**Also by Diana Lewis Jewell**

*Angel of Beauty, The Story of Dr. Erno Laszlo*
*Forever Beautiful with Rex,* by Rex Hilverdink, written by
     Diana Lewis Jewell
*Making Up by Rex,* by Rex Hilverdink, written by Diana Lewis Jewell
*Executive Style,* by Mary B. Fiedorek, written by Diana Lewis Jewell
*Anushka's Complete Body Makeover Book,* by Celestina Wallis and
     Anna Blau, written by Diana Lewis Jewell
*Lisanne, A Young Model,* by Betsy Cameron, written by
     Diana Lewis Jewell

# GOING GRAY,

## LOOKING GREAT!

### the modern woman's guide to unfading glory

## DIANA LEWIS JEWELL

PHOTOGRAPHS BY PETER FREED

A FIRESIDE BOOK

PUBLISHED BY SIMON & SCHUSTER    New York    London    Toronto    Sydney

FIRESIDE
Rockefeller Center
1230 Avenue of the Americas
New York, NY 10020

FIRESIDE and colophon are registered trademarks
of Simon & Schuster, Inc.

For information regarding special discounts for bulk purchases,
please contact Simon & Schuster Special Sales at 1-800-456-6798
or business@simonandschuster.com

Designed by Bonni Leon-Berman

Manufactured in the United States of America

10   9   8   7   6   5   4   3   2   1

Library of Congress Cataloging-in-Publication data is available

ISBN 0-7432-4680-2

To David Lloyd Jewell, who can always turn gray into a silver lining.

# contents

# contents

# a note to readers

THE INFORMATION contained in this book is meant to provide an overview of all the many "looking great" options available today. Written with the conviction that an informed beauty consumer is a better beauty consumer, it is in no way intended to be prescriptive. Any time you consider the use of chemicals on, or near, your face, or any cosmetic procedure, it is always advisable to consult with your doctor, dentist, or hair and skincare professionals. The author and publisher expressly disclaim responsibility for any adverse effects that may arise from the use or application of any products or procedures described herein.

# introduction

The enthusiasm for this book has been tremendous. Unexpectedly so. From the first moment I started talking to women about it, I was urged to do the book, begged to. "Oh, you *have* to," women would say. "There's nothing for us." Very often, if a man was within earshot, he'd asked me to put a chapter in for him, as well. "What about guys? We go gray!" Not one person said they were afraid of gray, or tired of being gray, or dreading going gray. They were proud of their streaks, their pure silver crop, their blend of black and white. They wanted to share tips, learn techniques, and simply go on record saying that gray hair can be beautiful. And they wanted other women to know this, to take delight in whatever stage of graying they were in. Writing this book became a commitment to them. And to myself, old enough and gray enough to face the decision that literally millions of boomers are facing every day. To gray or not to gray? That, indeed, is the question.

But, just as our generation put liposuction, plastic surgery, BOTOX, and anti-aging products on the map, we want to gray youthfully and beautifully. We want to be just as sexy, just as chic, just as fashionable as we have always been. We know it's going to take some work, but we're used to that. We're just not sure what to do, exactly. Commitment and encouragement aside, I had a mission with this book. I wanted to tell women how to add life, sparkle, and, yes, color if need be, to make every stage of going gray absolutely gorgeous. In essence, how to keep their gray, and their cool, too.

Buoyed at this prospect, I found myself one morning in an elevator with a young-looking gray-haired woman. She had her hair tightly pulled back off of her face and banded into a ponytail. There it was, particularly pretty in its melding of silvery tones, but it didn't look pretty. It looked old. The interesting thing was, *she* didn't look old. I guessed midthirties. Her face, without much makeup at all, appeared to be unlined. Her skin was glowing. Her eyes were a bright clear blue, and she was not wearing glasses. Must be genetically early, I thought. She noticed I was staring.

"I'm looking at your hair," I said. "I'm writing a book about gray hair, and I was wondering how you like having hair that color."

Her blue eyes brightened even more. The elevator continued its climb, and she wanted to talk.

"Oh, I love it," she said. And then she got a funny, frightened look on her face. Her eyes darted around the elevator, making sure we were alone. Then she lowered her tone.

"Of course, I use something to color it when I go for job interviews. It just doesn't work when you walk in with gray hair."

"Why? You're obviously young. You can't mean you're facing age discrimination already."

"I'm fifty-six," she admitted.

I was stunned. But maybe her actual age coupled with her gray hair was enough to do her in. At least, in her own mind. And then I looked at the way she wore it again. She was giving in to gray, and to age. Her only defense was to hide it. To pull it back, to take it away from her face, and to color it for job interviews. The elevator reached my floor, and I stepped out. She still wanted to talk, almost desperately. She held the door open.

"It's a shame because everybody gets old," she said, surprisingly vehemently. "*Everybody*. I don't see why—" and then someone else got in the elevator. She couldn't hold the door open anymore. She couldn't talk about it anymore. As the door was closing, I saw her give a small smile, a shrug, and a secretive little wave. It's just between us girls, all right?

Wow, I thought. My first encounter with a woman frightened of her own hair. And then I remembered where I was. I was in the building that houses Hearst Publications, purveyors of magazines that extol youth and beauty. Could she be afraid of her own gray because she worked for publications that were afraid of gray? No, that couldn't be true, I thought. Weren't there all those "How to Look Great at any Age" articles?

I had gotten off on the *Harper's Bazaar* floor. In the reception area was a giant blowup of their latest issue. Michelle Pfeiffer was on the cover. A woman who *admits* to being forty-four. A ripe old age, in cover girl chronology. And, interestingly, the age at which many women are nearing a pretty healthy level of graying. You couldn't tell it from Michelle. She was gloriously sun-streaked blonde. Fine, that's one thing you can do about gray. But I was wondering about the other women, the women who want to look glamorous and let their gray show. And maybe wear a black leather dress, like Michelle. Was the magazine that put a forty-four-year-old movie star on its cover going to speak to them?

I flipped through the pages. This issue had a "Hair Special" section. Oh good, I thought, let's see. Small little pictures of "Best Tressed" celebrities yielded nary a gray streak. But then there were three full-page beauty shots. One nineteen-year-old celebrity brunette, one nearing-thirty socialite blonde, and there, there, on page 123, one glorious gray, Carmen, the irrefutably glamorous model who pioneered white hair by "deciding to stop coloring" nearly thirty years ago. Well, one out of three ain't bad. In fact, it's great. *Harper's Bazaar* gave one-third of their special section beauty faces to gray hair! How fabulous, how timely. How right for today, I thought.

Now, very few of us are going to gray like Carmen (much less look like the fine-featured beauty) without some kind of professional help, so I was more convinced than ever of the need for this book. Information is everything. It's one thing to put middle-aged women on the covers of fashion magazines. It's another thing to talk to them. To tell them the secrets of being fabulously gray. To delve into the care of persnickety hair, as well as the color. To talk makeup and fashion. Emotions and triumphs. Yes! I felt elated. The world *needs* this book.

Then I walked into my meeting with the marketing director, a pert, pretty blonde who, I would suspect from the fine lines around her eyes, was probably as adept at covering gray as I was. We were to discuss a possible promotion for the book. But just as we sat down, she launched into what sounded like an oft-delivered

# having a gray hair day?

**When does the moment of truth come?
And what will you do about it?**

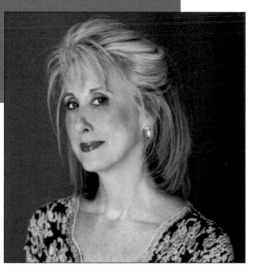

I used to think finding your first gray hair was one of those life experiences that were indelibly etched in your memory. You knew where you were and what you were doing when you saw it. It was for me. I was fourteen years old, it was a brilliant June day, and I was walking to the supermarket with my mother. Well, in front of my mother, actually, because who really walks *with* her mother at the age of fourteen? Suddenly, she said, "What is that in your hair?" I jumped around, thinking it was a bee, flapping my hands wildly around my head, "What, *what*? Get it out!" "Come here," she said, and began examining my scalp. Then I heard her give an amused laugh. "It seems to be rooted there." I was dying, something was growing on my head. I felt a small extraction. "You're going gray," she laughed, as she handed me a silvery shaft of hair. "My baby's going gray!" The only thing I felt was relief. Oh, that's all it is. I thought it was funny, because I knew I had years to go before I ever saw another one. That turned out to be true, although, for days after, I searched for more.

Maybe the trauma of thinking a foreign object was rooted to my head was the real reason I remember this so clearly. But I was surprised to find out that, for many women, finding their first gray hair was a non-event. Certainly not one they remember. I was prepared to write a dramatic opening to this book, describing the emotions, the fear of recognition, the shock. But not one woman I interviewed related such an experience. Most of them couldn't pin it down to a specific date, or even year. "I think I was twenty-three or twenty-seven, but I really don't remember." "I know we moved to Boston, because that's where I first started coloring my hair, but I don't know when it started to gray."

What *is* this? Denial? Doesn't seem to be. Whether the discovery of that first gray hair was accompanied by intense scrutiny, or mild curiosity, it just didn't stick. Especially if there was a significant lag time between the first grays, and a multitude. Women do remember when they first noticed a significant amount of graying in their hair. The moment they admitted, maybe to no one but themselves, that they were actually "going gray."

## poliosis. sounds like a disease, doesn't it?

*"She was so young and vibrant, and then, at about the age of thirty-five, she developed poliosis."*

Poor thing? Not really. All that happened to this woman was a pigment slowdown. Poliosis comes from the Greek word *polios*, which means gray. Poliosis is simply the graying of hair, sometimes in localized patches. It's not an affliction; it may be an anomaly, but it is usually a normal physiological process, programmed by genetic code. Nothing more, nothing less.

Of course, until only very recently, there were those who approached depigmentation with dread. But attitudes are changing as the population changes. More and more of us, it seems, have poliosis. Ever since 1996 when the first of the baby boomer generation neared the Big One, turning fifty, we've been told that someone turns fifty every seven seconds. Seemed rather alarming at the time, but so far the numbers have tallied up to almost 16 million women in their fifties, and over 43 million between the ages of forty and sixty-four, according to the U.S. Census Bureau's 2000 statistics. Add 21.5 million more, for those in their thirties (when many women begin to gray), and it's safe to say, "There's a whole lotta grayin' goin' on!"

**so now what?** But now it's time to decide what to do about it. If, like many women today, you don't want to begin, or continue, a monthly schedule of temporary, semipermanent, permanent, bleaching, or highlighting processes, this book is for you. If you feel you've lost your color "identity," this book is for you. If you want to feel your hair is as glorious as it ever was, and you want to try everything under the sun to keep it that way, this book is for you. If you want to learn how to be a whole new you, this book is for you. We're not talking about growing old gracefully, taking the gray one day (one strand) at a time. We're talking about Going Gray, Looking Great! From this moment on.

**making the decision** There's no gray area when it comes to deciding about going gray. You are either going to color the fading strands, or you aren't. It's really that simple. Deciding to use color complicates it a bit. How you use color, what type of color you use, is another story. You'll find out more about that later in the book, but first—to gray or not to gray, that *is* the question.

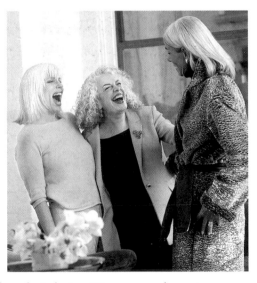

Deciding to go gray is not like deciding what color to paint the bedroom. It's easier. For many women, it's not a decision; it's a conviction. If their hair wants to lose its pigment, they're not going to stop it. Or make it turn a color it never was in its natural life. Are these "purists" a distinct minority? Surprisingly not. According to an AARP survey, 53 percent of women over fifty color their hair; 47 percent do not. Pretty close. And that doesn't include the women in their thirties and forties who have already decided to go with the gray.

Reasons for staying gray are as firmly rooted as reasons women have for coloring their hair. They may be different reasons, but they have the same strong note of resolve:

- I want to be me.
- I would never put chemicals on my hair.
- My hair is (dry) (fragile) (thinning), and I don't want to harm it.
- I think it's unique.
- I can't make a commitment to a regular coloring regimen.
- I hate the idea of roots.
- I love the freedom.
- I just like it.
- It's easier.
- I don't have time to fuss with color.

However expressed, the motivation to gray seems to fall into three camps: hair health, individuality, and simplicity. For some women, it's a little of each. For others, it's an issue they don't want to deal with at all.

> "I haven't even looked into dyeing it, and I don't want to. I mean, why? That whole fascination with every little gray hair is beyond me. I just don't want to know about it."
> **Dara Roche, producer, CBS morning news**

If you look again at the reasons for not coloring gray hair, you'll see that they're the same reasons women have for not coloring their hair when they aren't gray. So what's the difference? What does gray add to the equation? *Disorientation:* It's new to you. It's like nature adding a color to your hair, whether you have the time for the appointment or not. It *is* you and it *is* natural, but it's not the "you" you've always seen in the mirror. And it's easy, all right, but

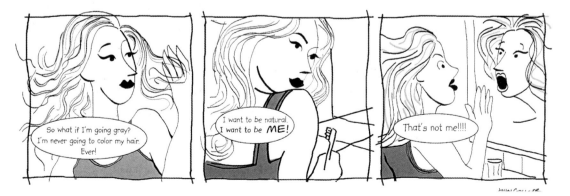

it may take a different kind of care. No, it's not the same as deciding to color your hair or not when you have a full head of vibrant color. You've got to think about this one.

## getting to the root of your decision Why do

some women decide to go with what nature gives them, and others refuse? Vanity? Fear of aging? Professional pressure? Peer pressure? All of these things may come into play, of course, but they are all a part of what clinical psychologist Patricia Moscou calls "Impression Management." Far from implying an unhealthy obsession with appearance, impression management is the way you choose to present yourself. An affirmation of the "inner you," to be sure, but projected in a way that confirms the way you see yourself.

According to Dr. Moscou, it has to do with your relation to the rest of the world. "You have a definition of yourself," she says, "but you may not want to reveal everything. And so you have to create some distance between yourself and others." This distance is the result of careful editing; you keep what you want others to see; you discard, camouflage, or change what you don't. The process can cause some dissonance, however. If what you reflect belies who you are inside, your own opinion of yourself, you will not be comfortable with your image. It's a total disconnect between what's inside and what's outside.

Chazz Levi, a florist, event planner, and occasional model, used a variety of hair colors to adapt to new environments, kind of like the adaptive coloring that animals take on to avoid predators. But she certainly didn't blend in. "I started to gray at eighteen," she says. "And I've been every color imaginable since then. I call it geographic coloring, because I did henna in India, a dark black/brown in Italy, and purple in the East Village. I let my son pick out the shade, and he chose his favorite color. Then I went to navy. It was quite a look. But I got to the point where I didn't know what color it was underneath anymore. So I started going lighter and lighter, just to see what I had. A little before my fortieth birthday, I saw I was white. And that's when I stopped coloring it."

# "White was my 40th birthday gift to myself."

Gray hair is a statement about yourself, and if you feel good about that statement, there will be little anxiety. You are saying to the world, "This is me. Take me the way I am." But what if you don't choose to say that? Does that mean you are hiding something? Does it mean you are not comfortable with yourself? No to both counts. It may mean that the "inner you" isn't gray at all. It is not how you see yourself; therefore, it is not how you want others to see you. You are being completely honest with yourself. There's no dissonance whatsoever.

The only time anxiety enters into the picture, according to Dr. Moscou, is when a woman can't figure out her inner self. "If you don't know who you are," she says, "you can make poor choices."

While finding the inner self can be a daunting journey, sometimes requiring professional help, Dr. Moscou suggests a simple exercise that is well worth trying. It could give you a clue to whether gray is right for you or not.

## getting to know your inner adult Imagine

concentric circles of people around you. At the outer ring are complete strangers. The ring closest to you is your family. The center ring is you. Now think:

1. **Strangers.** These are the people you pass on the street. You don't know any of them. They don't know you. *Do you care* if they see you as a gray-haired woman?
2. **Friends.** Your closest, and even your most competitive, friends are discussing your hair. *Do you care* what they say about the gray?
3. **Employers.** You've had a good track record on your job. Employers respect your skills and the image you project. *Do you care* if they respond negatively to your gray hair?
4. **Family.** Your loved ones may be all for it, or completely against it. Of course

you care about them, but this isn't about that. *Do you care* what they think about your hair?

5. **You.** What do you really think about seeing yourself as a gray-haired woman? What if there were no other circles around you, no other people who could influence your decision?

When you break it down like this, you can clearly gauge your own reaction to opinions of others. It is suddenly not a faceless, nameless mass of people staring at your hair. Each group may have a different reaction. And you will weight their reactions according to the importance of the group to you. Every woman will evaluate this differently. Only you can figure it out for yourself.

## it doesn't hurt to ask
While you're coming to terms with how much you care about what people think, it may also be helpful to hear what those close to you have to say. A "beauty mentor" is a great idea; and it can be a friend, relative, or business associate. Movie producer Amy Robinson listened to a friend, someone who was quite aware of the power of gray hair: Richard Gere. "We were sitting at lunch one day, and he said, 'How come my hair is all gray, and your hair is all brown?' I think he really inspired me to go gray," she says. "Richard has become comfortable in his own skin, and with his own hair. It's part of what his identity is as a person. And he's certainly very youthful with his gray hair." What better mentor can a girl have than the guy who made gray hair sexy? Most of us, of course, are not going to sit and chat with Richard Gere, but look around you. There are people who can, and will, give you very good advice. Sometimes you just have to ask. Sometimes you don't.

"I have a friend who is always trying to get me to color my hair," says real estate agent Rita Citrin, a woman who has enjoyed every moment of the graying process. "And she always comes up with different angles when I say no. She'll say I could put a little darker color in the back, or just put some highlights in the front. She's always on me about this."

# i don't care what anybody thinks. but . . .

Let's say other people's opinions are not part of the equation. You've dealt with that; it's fine. What is it, then, that makes you feel unsure?

"It's a little like adolescence," Dr. Moscou says. "You are becoming a different person, if only visually. If this suddenly happens overnight, it could be traumatic." Fortunately, graying is a process. You have time to adjust, and to explore your feelings. Unfortunately, like adolescence, it hits you just about the same time your hormones are shifting. Your skin is aging. Your body is changing. And your confidence may be at an all-time low. All of the issues of aging are staring you smack in the face. Now you turn gray.

So maybe that's what the inner you is dealing with. It may have more to do with fear of aging than fear of graying. Graying is the tip of the iceberg. It may cause you to think about lost youth, decreasing vitality, even mortality. It's serious business, when you think about it. The point is, think about it. Know your reasons. Know your fears. Know your reaction to what others may think. Then, and only then, can you make the decision that is right for you.

# husbands, lovers, and kids

Many women tell me the encouragement to keep their gray came from their husbands. "I wish you would just let it go gray," they'd say. (Let's not even *think* they were looking at the salon bills!) But what about the ones who just aren't comfortable with a gray-haired wife? Could it be the old-by-association worry? "If my wife is old enough to have gray hair, what does that make me?" Could it be the Oedipus-in-reverse conflict? A man may feel a graying wife will remind him of his mother. Could it be he finds only young women sexy and attractive? Don't assume anything. Try to find out his real reasons for resistance.

Your husband may still see you as the "girl" he married. While that seems very romantic, it's a bit restrictive. You are not the same girl. You have, with all of life's experiences together, matured into the woman you are today. If he is keeping you in a time warp, it's time to talk! Growing together is a wonderful, crazy, remarkable journey. But it is difficult to move into the future while hanging on to the past. Perhaps giving *him* "permission" to go gray is a good place to embark.

Finally, there's the fear factor. Husbands tend to think that everything is going to change when your hair color changes. You'll let yourself go. You won't be interested in looking appealing (or being appealing!). First your hair goes gray. Then you'll start wearing gunny sacks. You won't, of course. And once he sees that you're maintaining your own persona, he'll quickly stop worrying about stereotypes.

If no amount of reassurance works, tell your husband you're simply trying it out—like any hair color. But give it your best shot. Make sure you're the most fabulous gray you can be. If nobody likes it, including yourself, you can always go back.

**sexy or not?** For every man who has his doubts about gray, there's another one who thinks it's sexy. Absolutely! There are husbands who love it, boyfriends who wouldn't want you any other way, and younger men who will follow you anywhere. Admittedly, the younger you go gray, the less it is perceived as an aging issue. A man sees gray hair on a twenty- or thirty-year-old woman as an anomaly, unusual enough to be "edgy" and exciting. But even if gray comes to you later in life, there are men aplenty who will see you as more attractive than ever. "I'm getting that thing with men now—that chromosome thing that attracts them to blondes," says Chazz Levi. "I'm beautiful now."

So what's this about younger men? It's definitely not a "mother thing," I've been assured by many women. Younger men are attracted to the confidence and competence of older women, and gray hair can act like a pheromone, a chemical signal that attracts animals of the same species. It sends a maturity signal instantly. "Younger men like older women," explains Chazz. "They say we know ourselves better, so we're not as needy. Men don't like needy women."

But younger men aren't the only ones who appreciate gray. A midfifties woman said her husband was always "proud to show her off," pre-gray. Well, she's gray now, still looking fabulous, and her husband, who had "twinges" about the whole idea, is still proud to show her off. The point is, if you were sexy before, you'll still be sexy. If you were attractive before, you'll still be attractive. If you were vivacious and fun to be around before, you'll still be vivacious and fun. Your personality isn't going to change. Neither is the attitude you have about yourself. The way you carry yourself. The weight you maintain. Your own sense of style. "We all lock and load at a certain age," says Chazz. "We think of ourselves as twenty-four or twenty-eight, and that sticks with us in our attitudes." This isn't necessarily a bad thing. It's

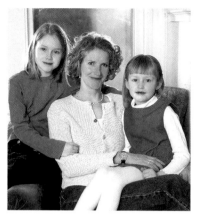

what gets us through graying—and aging—with our inner youth intact.

Of course, while we may be somewhere in our twenties inwardly, we're walking around in the body of an older woman. Producer Amy Robinson is a bit more realistic about it. "As you get older, somehow you get more anonymous, whether you have gray hair or not," she says. "Face it, you're not the twenty-three-year-old who gets whistled at. But it's about how you see yourself." If you see yourself with the right attitude, others will see it, too. No matter what your age. Keep your gray, put on a smile, and you may be the fifty-year-old woman who gets whistled at!

Gray and kids? Jennie Bernard proves it's a beautiful mix.

Women who gray early are often worried about their children's reactions to a gray-haired mommy. Will the kids like it? Will they be embarrassed? Will they think I'm getting old? These are adult concerns, but they don't seem to occur to children at all. Many women report that their kids were all for it. One forty-something woman told me she tried everything but "repotting" her hair when she started to turn gray. It was her children who told her to *please* let it go natural. She did. She's happy; they're happy.

Kid-incentive worked for Carmine Fuentes's mother, as well. "My sister and I used to ask our mom to stop coloring her hair. We wanted it to look natural," she remembers. Their mother gave in, had beautiful white hair, and today, Carmine has the same.

Young children find an interesting advantage to Mom being gray. Chazz Levi, who stopped coloring her hair just before her daughter turned eight, reports that her little girl loved it because "she could find me in a crowd. I was always easy to spot."

As with adults, children's reactions can be unpredictable. Alice Feder, of

Chatham, Massachusetts, the mother of a seven-year-old, says she is sometimes mistaken for her daughter's grandmother by her school friends. "I may be ten years older than most of the mothers here, but I'm not that old! I think children automatically associate gray hair with their grandmas," she laughs. "It doesn't really bother me. I tell them, 'No, I'm her mother, and this is just my hair color.' "

**one more thing: the mother factor** We know the age at which your hair stops producing pigment is preprogrammed in your genes. But your mother may have a lot more to do with your decision to stay gray than you think. Look back at how she handled her graying. Are you dealing with it the same way?

Lawyer Amy Trakinski, who started graying in college, and decided to go with it, remembers: "When we were kids, my mother would come out of the bathroom with those plastic gloves on, and every time her hair was a different shade, because she colored it herself. But when she went into real estate, and came into her own as a professional woman, she started getting great haircuts, and that's when she let it grow in. And she always looked fabulous."

> "I didn't realize until we started talking about it how big an influence she was on me, and my staying gray."

Liz Cullumber, a silver-haired model you would recognize by her signature short cut, didn't find out until later in life how beautiful her mother looked with gray hair. "I started turning gray at nineteen, but never knew if it ran in my family or not because I was adopted. In those days, the natural thing to do was color it; you'd go to your hairdresser, and he'd say, 'Oh, this is making you look old.' So I was covering it more and more."

"And then I found my birth mother at the age of forty-one, and when I met her, her hair was completely white and lovely, and I just liked it."

This can work in reverse as well. Let's say your mother colored her hair until a significant life change. Perhaps the death of your father, perhaps the point at which she retired. She "gave up" on color as she was giving up on life as she knew it. It sends a signal many daughters heed: Gray is a sign of giving up.

Amy Robinson's mother sent a different signal. She went back to work in her sixties and refused to color her hair. "It was the beginning of women's lib, of women being who they are," Amy noted, "and I think she used this to set herself apart." Her mother, Estelle, confirmed this on her eighty-second birthday. "I just didn't want to look like a suburban wife," she remembered. It wasn't a case at all of giving up. Estelle kept regular salon appointments every week. But color was not an option.

A mother's influence can have the opposite effect. JoAnne Pinto, who spotted her first gray hairs at the age of ten and was noticeably streaked with gray at fourteen, used to watch her mother dye her hair. She made her decision there and then.

"I would look at my mom on dye days and think, This is nuts. It takes too long; it smells bad. I will never do it, no matter what."

Being born the daughter of a world-famous beauty doesn't make a difference in the way you perceive the coloring process. Sculptor Mia Fonssagrives Solow, whose mother was Lisa Fonssagrives, the iconic model of the 1950s, never followed in her mother's footsteps to the beauty salon. After Mia started to gray in her twenties (quite suddenly, after an appendectomy operation), she never, ever colored her hair.

"My mother was a great beauty. And every week, she would be in the beauty parlor, getting her hair colored whatever shade it needed to be. It seemed like such a waste of time."

Deborah Aiges, a former vice president and creative director of Random House Publishing Group, balked against her mother's example, as well. She remembers, "My mom was very put together—makeup, clothing, accessories—and she wanted me to be, too. I was a little more relaxed than that."

"But until the day she died, she thought I should be coloring my hair."

Why do mothers care so? It's a little like husbands. Yes, they may honestly feel their daughters would look younger without the gray. ("And get a husband," Rita Citrin adds.) But more than one woman said concern over aging was more about the mother. "My mother said she felt older just looking at me!" reported violinist Setsuko Nagata Ikeda, who started noticing "more and more" gray hair at the age of forty-one.

"For a while, I dyed it for her. If it weren't for her, I don't think I would have started coloring it."

We've all been brought up to listen to our mothers. But, along the way, we learn to filter their advice through our own sense of self. At critical times, however, it's natural to fall back on established patterns, and "Mother knows best" seems the

"Gray hair can be elegant. Inviting. What I am attracted to is a woman who smiles. One who is a happy person; I rarely notice hair color. Gray or not is not a huge factor in attractiveness. But I don't like 'blue.' "
*Greg, 51, developer, Erie, Pennsylvania*

"I think my wife looks more beautiful than ever. I love her gray hair. That's part of our life together. I would hate for her to dye it."
*André, 46, publisher, Hastings-on-Hudson, New York*

"The sexiest thing about a woman with classic beauty is the wisdom of her gray."
*Rus, 35, teacher, Colton, California*

"I see personality. Hair color is secondary."
*John, 47, attorney, Orange, California*

"Like the lustre on fine pearls, silver hair is a woman's patina."
*Christopher, 56, attorney, Chicago, Illinois*

"I think it's hot. One, because it shows a woman has the confidence to wear her hair any color she wants. And two, because chances are good she's an ex-hippie chick."
*John, 52, art director, New York, New York*

# café au gray

**A roundtable discussion. Women tell all.**

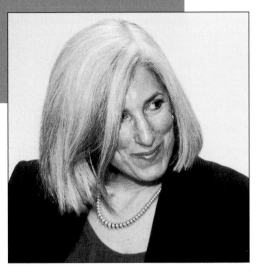

At six P.M., twelve women converged upon the Minardi Salon in New York. From their chic, well-groomed looks, you might have assumed they were keeping their standard after-work appointments. But, if you looked again, you would be aware that most of them had gray hair. A variety of shades, to be sure, but undeniably gray.

They were there for a reason. They had been asked to talk about going gray, being gray, *dealing* with gray. Women from a variety of professions and lifestyles. Women at various stages of gray. An interesting group. Among them, a designer of household products, a television news writer, two psychologists, a special events planner for nonprofit organizations, a horticulturist, a massage therapist, a financial adviser, a flight attendant, an actress, a consultant, and a full-time homemaker. Two of them were still adding color to mask the appearance of gray. Two of them were enhancing their gray with special color effects. The rest were letting nature take its glorious course.

They were there because a book on Going Gray, Looking Great! must begin with the women who are doing it, living it, looking it. They wanted to talk about being gray. I wanted to listen. And to ask the questions women everywhere wanted to ask. Particularly women who are facing the "to be or not to be" decision about going gray. What is it like? How do you feel about it? What are you doing to maintain it?

Going gray, of course, is a process. One that starts with the first gray hair. That chilling little portent of things to come can pop up at any time, for any number of reasons. Not all of them associated with your body's aging clock. While the standard age of onset is fixed at midthirties, this group proved otherwise. A few discovered that startling little shaft in their teens, one in her midforties, but most spotted their first gray hair in their late twenties. Some were very specific about the exact date, "I was twenty-seven, and in San Francisco." Others were, surprisingly, vague. This presumably monumental occurrence was simply a non-event. Many had to guess at their age. Some admitted, frankly, "I don't really remember."

Chris, who is highlighting her grays away, grew up with a pure white "birthmark streak." It had been around since she was ten or twelve. At some point, it "started spreading out a lot."

Pat, whose long gray hair still looks blond to others, considered herself lucky to go gray in her early twenties. "My father had gone gray in college, and my mother at twenty-one. So I thought I had done very well."

The age at which a woman finally knows that the renegade white strands have coalesced into an obvious shade of gray occurs later. Patricia, who spotted her first gray hair in her late twenties, was significantly gray before the age of thirty-five. Today, she has the kind of perfect, smooth, pure white hair any woman would willingly go gray for. Most of the women, however, didn't perceive themselves as graying until their midforties, or later. One or two placed the date closer to fifty.

Carol, with a short cap cut so beautifully striated with shades of silver that people were always asking her who did her frosting, looked in the mirror at the age of fifty-nine and realized, "Oh my God, it's just gray. It's not streaky, It's not anything else, it's just *gray*." She added with a smile, "And that was fine."

It's at this point that many admitted to doing something about it. "I was forty-three," said Leni, "and I decided it was time for Loving Care." The others nodded and giggled in recognition. Today, Leni is a single-process strawberry blonde, believing her skin too "ghost white" to go well with gray or white hair.

Sherrill also went the Loving Care route, then switched to something else. Trying one product after another, in search of a natural look, held little appeal. She has just recently decided to let it grow in, but she's still not sure of her commitment. Although her gray is not contrasting unattractively with her medium-brown hair, she has a wait-and-see attitude. "I'm not convinced yet," she admitted.

Perhaps this same indecision caused some women to hold out before coloring their hair. They didn't react to the first grays, or even to the ensuing "grayness" of their hair.

Angela, with just the beginnings of gray peppering her scalp-short, tight curls, the hair of an Afro-Caribbean heritage, is an early holdout. "I haven't done anything yet," she said.

"I didn't do anything about it until I turned totally white. First I streaked it black in front, and then the rest was white," said Peri, a petite woman with a short crop of black hair and a striking white streak sweeping through her bangs. "But then I decided I looked old from behind. That's the worst place to look old. So now I'm doing the reverse."

Anne-Renée, a woman whose hair is a sleek, steely charcoal, also waited to color her hair. "I waited until I couldn't stand it anymore. Then I took a bottle, and said, 'I can do this myself,' and it worked for a while. But then I decided I needed some help. So I started having it dyed a soft, dark brown."

"I did henna," remembered Marilyn, her glistening ringlets a profusion of silvery shades, "and then the regular dye stuff. And more recently, glosser, which is a low-peroxide product. And all that was very nice; I was blonde. But then, when so much came in, I said '*Hmmmmm*, I like it!' "

Ilene had the same positive reaction. Her lively, pure-white bob shows no trace of what she had put it through. "At first I warmed it up, and that was fine. But it was going on for years. I had a braid halfway down my back, and I suddenly saw it was three colors—gunmetal gray from the top down, then brown, then oxidized. So I went to my hairdresser and said, 'Let's do something.' "

Marilyn sympathized. "I had that seven-layer thing going on. Like a seven-layer cake. My hair was a cake."

Ellen approached color from another angle. "For me, the decision was not to go gray, but whether to color my hair. And I find color an enormous commitment.

lady. So, according to them, I had to be blond. I was more comfortable with gray hair than blond, but that was their mentality."

**Q. We've talked about other people being afraid of your gray hair, but now, what were you afraid of? If anything?**

**Carol:** "Up until the age of forty-nine, my hair was so long I could sit on it. I decided the last thing I wanted to be was this little gray-haired old lady with a bun in the back, and lots of lovely antique combs and pins. So I kept snipping and snipping and snipping, and yeah, there's a change that happens there."

**Anne-Renée:** "I think one of the things that concerned me was being on television. It was growing out, and I wasn't coloring it. So I cut it shorter, and then a little shorter, until finally, I said to my hairdresser, 'Cut it all off, I only want to see gray.' And it was wonderful! It was like coming of age; it felt great."

**Ilene:** "We have no role models. All the gray-haired women we know were all those blue-haired ladies with spit curls. That's scary to me. I don't want to be that, and I know when I'm walking down the street and people see me, that's what's running through their minds. Somehow there's that image. And the position that I take is: 'That's *your* problem.'"

**Carol:** "I think we're the first gray-haired generation that's not invisible."

**Ilene:** "That's the key word."

**Carol:** "Older women have always been invisible. At fifty, you sort of fade out. Your hair color, everything. We're not doing that."

**Ilene:** "But it's a struggle, every day. Just to make yourself heard, make yourself seen. Not be somebody's mother."

**Carol:** "And not be patronized."

**Angela:** "I'm more hopeful about looking totally gray, now, but hitting the work force may bother me."

**Ellen:** "Although in my industry [financial], that's changing now. All of a sudden, people with gray hair are appreciated because of the experience it represents. You know, they've lived through good markets and bad markets, and that's now attractive. Actually that's the kind of people you want dealing with clients."

**Anne-Renée:** "We're talking about credibility. And I think, for me in psychology, the gray hairs just add credibility. It really feels good—I have thirty years of experience. Here I am!"

**Q. How do you all feel now? Now that you're more comfortable with your appearance? Or are you?**

**Ilene:** "I think, like a lot of you, I felt myself liberated. Suddenly, it was me! And I finally stopped looking in windows as I passed, saying, 'Who is that person?' "

**Ellen:** "You know, it is a youth-driven society, but I think there's more acceptance of [gray hair] now. I also think it has to do with how you carry yourself. If you carry yourself like someone old, then it doesn't matter what color hair you have. And I try not to do that. Actually, I'm younger than my daughter would like me to be."

**Patricia:** "You have to be brave and strong in a world that treasures youth, that overvalues youth."

**Ilene:** "The aging thing is what you carry in your head."

As we switched from personal and professional concerns to hair management, the women seemed a little less forthcoming. Could it be that gray hair presented no particular problems at all? This was hard to believe, but when asked how their hair had changed when it started to gray, say 20 to 30 percent gray, most mentioned it was "coarser, thicker." Some noted that their hair was "more fragile" or "a little softer, but otherwise the same." Some said it became drier. A few said they noticed no change at all. Ellen's hair, however, started doing surprising things. "Mine grew straight out from my head. It was not attractive."

If the hair had changed, in some way, you might think that manageability would become a problem. A big no, all around. It didn't. Some said coloring it helped, others said their hair was actually easier to manage. Ellen turned to chemical straightening to solve her tricky sticking out problem, but nothing else was needed.

As far as dryness goes, most wouldn't admit to it being exclusively the "fault" of graying. Peri pointed out that "everyone our age" seems to have dry hair, whether it's from coloring it, or from other hormonal changes. Gray hair was not the only culprit.

Nor was it blamed for thinning hair. Only two women noticed that problem, but again, chalked it up to "postmenopausal" or "stress."

It was time to talk about products. These women had discovered what worked for them, what didn't, and they didn't want to hold back.

**Marilyn:** "I use shampoos for either gray and colored hair. I have for years."

**Carol:** "If I use shampoos for gray hair, it's guaranteed to just dull my hair out and make me look dead. It makes my hair look dead."

**Chris:** "I balance every other shampoo with a clarifying shampoo. One's for color, one's regular, otherwise it gets very flat and heavy."

**Anne-Renée:** "You should use different shampoos, every time."

Suddenly, names were being called out. A barrage of names and products. Everyone had a favorite something-or-other, but not a big-deal care plan.

Except when it came to that funny yellow cast that gray hair can get.

**Carol:** "One of the things that you have to watch for, at least I do, is certain shampoos turn your hair yellow and make a bad situation worse."

There were nods of agreement all around. You'll learn in a later chapter that it's not shampoos that turn gray hair yellow, but what this group revealed readily was the solution: Many used a "blue" shampoo, from time to time. Their favorites? Aveda's Blue Malva, Clairol's Shimmer Lights, and John Frieda's #2 Shampoo.

Staying clear of smokers and polluted cities was another answer. But short of staying in an air-filtered room, how was a woman to keep her silvery locks shining? I suspected good conditioners, but I was wrong. Exactly half of the group didn't use conditioners at all.

**Sherrill:** "I don't even use conditioner anymore."

**Chris:** "I don't either, it makes it too soft. Flat and lifeless."

**Anne-Renée:** "As course as my hair might be, it just takes all the life out of it."

**Angela:** "I don't use a conditioner either. Just whatever I use to moisturize my body, I use on my hair. And I haven't had a problem."

**Pat:** "My hair is like bunny fur, so I don't need to use conditioner for detangling. If I put a bobby pin or anything into it, it slides right out!"

So what did they use to keep their gray hair lively? Sherrill thought her shine came from the absence of product, from not using conditioners or anything else. Chris relied on the conditioners already in coloring products; "They keep your hair in pretty good shape." The others opted for topical polishers.

**Peri:** "I use Vitapointe; I just rub it on my hands and on my hair, and it looks shiny. Even if I went all white, it would still look shiny."
**Marilyn:** "I wish I could find Palmitex. It used to make my hair glisten, like shoe polish. It's green, and I remember the smell. It was just delicious."

Shea butter got a few votes, too, for an occasional moisturizing treatment. But, clearly, conditioners were not essential to control hair, or help with manageability. That left styling aids.

**Q. Do any of you use more, or less styling aids than you did before you went gray?**

A smattering of women said "More" and an equal number said "None." Yes, Ellen had had her hair chemically straightened, and Sherrill used a curling iron to give her straight hair some body, but that seemed to be it. Tackle the major body problems and be done with it. "Well, you have to have a really good cut," Ilene stated, "and then I use the goo." Patricia was recently introduced to spike-making "hair wax" by her preteen son and found it worked to keep her long side sweep out of her eyes, but she doesn't use anything on a regular basis. Certainly a group without styling problems, but maybe only their hairdressers knew for sure. Certainly they had to discuss *some* problems with their stylists.

**Marilyn:** "Something in me makes me ask, 'Do you think we should do anything to it?' And he always says, 'No, it's too pretty.' I'm a fool for pretty."

Would they try any do-it-yourself color at home, now, to change things just a little? No. Unanimous. Would they try any color services at their salon? Two said

**Anne-Renée:** "I have to wear lipstick. There are days when I won't walk out of the house without lipstick because I look dead to myself."

**Ilene:** "I find myself going to the pinks and purples and deeper lipsticks and things I would not have worn before."

**Anne-Renée:** "I did find my face looked dead. Here, I loved my hair, and my face looked dead. So I had to change everything."

**Ilene:** "We're redefining beauty. It's all unknown territory. We have to get rid of preconceived attitudes and ideas and figure out how do we respond to beauty. You have to reimagine yourself every day."

**Sherrill:** "I think that's one of the most important things—getting your skin color and your makeup to match your hair. Actually, I'd rather have that done than my hair done."

**Peri:** "Go to any department store, they'll fight over you."

**Sherrill:** "But the clothing, too, that's important."

So we talked about clothing. Did they change the colors in their wardrobe? And to what?

**Ilene:** "The blue reds. I suddenly was those winter colors, and I was dressing in all the wrong shades. All rusts and browns. Suddenly, it's all the silvers, magentas, and reds."

**Anne-Renee:** "You do look at colors differently. I haven't made too many changes, but I do wear more black, and I do wear reds. I never wore navy blues. But now look. White pearls. White earrings. It's gotta make my face look bright."

**Ellen:** "I went from black to black."

**Peri:** "I used to wear a lot of cream. Now I wear no cream at all. Or beige. It looks deadly."

**Chris:** "Camel's not a great color."

**Carol:** "And, God forbid, pale pink or pale blue."

**Peri:** "Bright pink is okay."

**Ilene:** "Fuchsia's good. Strong colors. All the purples and the magentas. Much more red, much more purple. Always."

**Marilyn:** "I stopped wearing beige. And I didn't do it premeditatively. I just noticed."
**Peri:** "It's all unconscious."

Even jewelry came in for a second appraisal. Several shouted out, "Silver, silver jewelry rather than gold." And, no dummies in this group, "Diamonds!"

These women had taken an active part in changing their appearance. They did not go gray passively. They thought it through, changed what needed to be changed, and liked the results. Still, still, if there were one thing they could change about their appearance, what would it be? What would be on their wish list?

**Ilene:** "Taller and thinner."
**Patricia:** "I'd be twenty-five again and know what I know now."
**Anne-Renée:** "Get rid of the cottage cheese."
**Leni:** "The whole face fixed."
**Angela:** "Not gain weight ever."
**Pat:** "Not to have wrecked my skin in the sun. It haunts me now."
**Ellen:** "I don't want to be thirty, but I'd like to have the body I had when I was thirty."
**Chris:** "Get rid of the wrinkles around my mouth."
**Marilyn:** "I'd like to be happy and thin. Usually I'm miserable when I'm thinner."
**Carol:** "Reline a couple of joints that don't quite work as well as they used to."
**Sherrill:** "I'd go for the thirty-year-old body."
**Peri:** "I'd be thinner, and never have to worry about gaining weight."

*None of these women said anything about changing their hair.*

Carol summed up what everybody was thinking, "We obviously don't want to, and it's not a major issue."

Going gray, being gray, is *not* a major issue. It's something you do well, you do right, and you enjoy. Or, as the panel pointed out, it's the easiest thing in the world to change.

# the color quandary

**There are so many ways to go gray, or not. Pick one.**

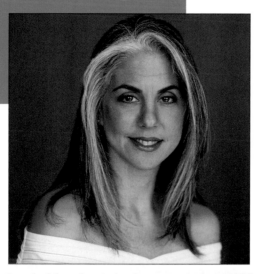

What color is your hair? If it's just starting to gray, you'll probably say blonde, brunette, black, or red. Or any one of the infinitesimal shadings within these color categories. Sandy blonde. Ashy brown. Auburn. Chestnut. If there's quite a bit of white streaking through it, you might say salt and pepper. Let's stop right there. Change the vocabulary a little, and it will change the perception. What's wrong with saying your hair is a mélange? A blonde mélange, a brunette mélange. It suggests a blending of tones, a mingling of shades—a much more beautiful way of thinking about gray.

And, while we're at it, why isn't gray included in the color dialogue? Why isn't it right up there beside blonde, brunette, and redhead? It may not be a birth color, and it may be due to the absence of pigment, but the effect is a true and honest overall *color*. We can dress it up a little bit. Just as we don't say "yellow" for blonde hair, we don't have to say gray. Our hair can be charcoal, sterling, pewter, silver, ice, snow, pearl. Why should blondes have all the fun?

Giving your gray a new name is more than semantics. It implies an attitude about gray, an acceptance of its natural beauty. Its pure, yes, *color*. It's time for the way we perceive gray to change. Time to strike the phrase "gray-haired old lady" from people's minds. Gray and age are no longer synonymous. Gray is simply a color *choice,* as Beth Minardi points out. A *color* choice.

## pick a color, any color
Like any color choice, gray takes some thought. And artistry. Maybe you make the choice to cover it. Or maybe you want to let it come in. Or maybe you want to enhance your gray, really make it pop. So many choices, so little direction.

Your friends tell you what they do. Your colorist tells you what he or she would do. But, before *you* do anything, it helps to know the vocabulary. One woman's "rinse" may be another woman's "glaze." And what's with the semi's and demi's, anyway? Here are the standard definitions for hair-coloring products:

**temporary**        Color that coats the hair shaft, then washes out. Good to "re-fresh" color, or try out a new shade.

**color rinse**       A semipermanent toner. Cuts down unwanted tones in the hair.

**demipermanent**     A color product that uses low-volume peroxide. Some have no ammonia. Color fades gradually, over eight-plus weeks, with no grow-out line.

**semipermanent**     Nonperoxide color that coats the hair. Also called glazes, stains, or washes because of translucent quality. Can optimize hair shine. Can cover gray and darken, but not lighten, hair. Washes out over four to six weeks.

**glaze**             A sheer, conditioning, semipermanent color gloss. Adds shine, but does stain hair.

**permanent**         Color that changes the natural hair color by penetrating shaft with peroxide. Reacts with the cortex of the hair to deposit or remove the color. Will not wash out. Roots will need to be re-touched every three to four weeks.

| | |
|---|---|
| **herbal** | Color treatment that is organic and natural. Coats the shaft without penetration. Has a conditioning and thickening effect, but may also dull hair due to buildup. The best known herbal color is henna. Caution: Turns hair without pigment orange. |
| **bleach** | A color-stripping product that oxidizes hair pigment with peroxide into a colorless form. Can weaken hair and increase porosity, leading to frizziness. |

**grabbing the bottle** The very first, very natural, reaction is to cover up the errant offenders. After all, your hair is predominantly the same color it has always been. The few white streaks are an aberration. The first bottle you might grab could be a color-enhancing shampoo. Its noninvasive pigments deposit color on the strand as you shampoo. At best, they're fine for a bit of brightening, and it's easy to select a shade near your own—nothing is that specific. Frédéric Fekkai has three, for instance: Baby Blonde, with chamomile and sunflower; Rio Red, with henna and ginger; and Brilliant Brown, with coffee bean, caramel, and henna. A color-enhancing shampoo does little more than refresh or "revive" your natural color, but it's a good pick-me-up, if your hair's got the first gray blahs. Next shampoo, it washes off.

At your salon, you may also find color-enhancing conditioners. Biolage has Earth Tones, a conditioner formulated in five nature-inspired shades. Developed to keep your salon color vibrant, these color-refreshing conditioners add a color boost to *any* hair (color-treated or not), making a minimal amount of gray seem to fade away.

If you want to do a bit more than simply liven up the color of your hair, the bottle you want is a temporary water-soluble rinse. Since these wash right out, they're a way to add color without making a commitment one way or the other. It's fun to experiment with color at this point, as long as it doesn't stick around. Before you decide to do anything serious, see how you look as an ashier brunette, a cooler blonde, a rich russet-haired beauty. Then, if you choose to cover your gray in a more permanent way, you'll know the direction in which to go.

applicator wand—just like your lip gloss. With a formula free of ammonia and per-oxide, ColorMark puts advanced color technology to work on your hair, gently conditioning it in the bargain. But the real news is, it sets in a minute, and can be brushed, sprayed, and styled without flaking out. The color disappears with your next shampoo, so it never interferes with your colorist's work, or your own redos. Just remember to wash it out before applying any permanent hair color. Select salons and specialty stores carry ColorMark, or you can find it by visiting www. colormarkpro.com, or calling 888-612-HAIR.

**Putting It On: The Art Of Applying Color** You have a world of coloring products from which to choose: lotions, creams, foams, gels, and nonammonia products. Which is right for you? Consider the length of your hair and the ease of application; lotions are better for even distribution over longer hair, easy-to-apply gels are great for short hair, creams offer moisturizing for higher shine, and nonammonia products create soft nuances without a strong lightening effect.

Whatever type of color product you choose, don't be surprised if your gray hair resists color stubbornly. Gray hair has a thicker cuticle, so the color may take longer to penetrate to the cortex. That's why it doesn't "grab" color. It also doesn't hold it. After a few shampoos, your hair can turn brassy.

When you apply your color, there are a few tricks that can help. Pay attention to the hairline, which is probably the grayest part of your hair. If you are using a dark color all over, the hairline can become black or drab. Just the opposite of what you want; color around the face is more flattering if it is a softer shade. Since you may have to leave your color on for the maximum recommended time, save the hairline area until last.

If you want to *match* a white streak, or a patch of gray that isn't pleasing, to your natural shade, choose a product that is *one* shade darker than your natural tone. The predominately pigmentless area will "take" one shade lighter than the product color, and you'll have a match. (Keep in mind, if you cover the whole head with this color, your natural color will go one step deeper, and you will have achieved a subtle blending, but not a match.) If you simply want to *blend* the white streak or area, it's easier to select one shade lighter than your natural color to begin with. That way, you haven't changed your natural shade, but you have nuanced the gray.

**Help, My Hair Won't Stay the Same Color!** Let's say you've found the perfect shade. It's a semipermanent color, and you expect it to last for a while. As it begins to wash out (and your white roots begin to show more and more), you're ready to apply it again. The second time, it's still the shade you like. The third time you apply it, you get a bit of a different result, and the forth time it's not the same as the third. Something starts happening to it. It's called color buildup. According to Beth Minardi, "If you use a semipermanent product, the first time it will wash out completely. But not the second time. The second time, maybe only 81 percent of it washes out. So color builds up eventually, and then just looks purply on the hair. You may never get the same results that pleased you the very first time, and you'll just keep trying and adding, and wondering why."

**Keep It Simple** Experts advise not tackling anything complicated, like a two-step coloring process, by yourself. It gets tricky to bring your overall hair color to the shade you desire, and the results have more to do with your underlying pigment tones than the actual product you select. Do you know your base tones? Don't say blonde, brunette, or red. Think yellow, violet, and blue. Surprising, but all natural hair color is composed of those tones. Dark brown hair has a lot of blue in it; yellow and violet cancel each other out. "When we bleach hair," says Carmine Minardi, co-owner and style director of the Minardi Salon, "the first thing we take out is the blue appearance, and then the hair turns red, then orange, then yellow, depending on how much blue is removed." And then there's the whole choice of toners, to add the final "color" you like, or offset shades you didn't bargain for. A gold-orange toner can neutralize a greenish cast; a green toner can turn orangy hair brown. It's all about tonal opposites on the color wheel. Do you feel you know enough about this to try it at home, alone, with rubber gloves?

## Choice 2: You're Going to Have Your Gray Covered Professionally.

Graying hair brings out the true artistry in a colorist. Most of the really good ones respect the nuancing and shadings of natural hair, and they use multiple techniques to achieve this.

A professional colorist knows that covering gray is a process, not a one-shot job. The first objective should be to make you just a little less gray, not to camou-

**Transition, Transition, Transition** "What's really wrong is to walk into my salon at ten in the morning and want to be gray two hours later when you walk out," Beth Minardi says. "It's bad for the hair, and it's much too drastic. You're going to walk into your next meeting, or social event, and someone is going to say 'Oh, what did you *do?*' and that's going to be the worst day of your life."

At the Minardi Salon, evolving into gray occurs over a period of six to eight appointments, with visits every four weeks or every three months. It allows the hair, and the woman, time to get used to it. "At some point, a woman will say, 'Stop—enough—that's enough gray.' Because there are so many degrees of gray. What we are doing is finding the level that works for her," says Beth.

Every woman is different. But if you want to know generally what can be done, let's book an appointment with Beth Minardi right now. Here are some "evolutions" she suggests:

**dark brunette:** "Most brunettes who have been graying for a while have been using something on their hair by the time they come to see me," Beth says. To correct this, she would begin by covering the gray with a nonammonia demicolor lighter than the one the woman has been using. Next, Beth would start to soften the color of selected strands around the face. This process would continue for three to four visits, evolving into a softer brown with several silvery strands around the face. The level of gray will increase until it reaches the grayness the woman wants.

**blonde:** A blonde should have a good eight to nine weeks of root growth before the process starts. Then Beth would use a very sheer, nonammonia blend that wouldn't make the pigmented hair lighter, but would make the gray strands blonde. Highlights would be added every three months. As the yellow in the woman's hair is minimized, it brings about more white. "She'll have a very nice, very soft shade of hair," says Beth.

**redhead:** "A successful redhead will have a harder time evolving into gray," Beth says, "but she can use gray to her advantage by simply shading it." The first thing Beth would do is to make the color softened and more muted. "If it's that bright shade of red, you've got to bring it down." Then, she would stroke in bold and subtle streaks of the palest blonde, a white blonde at the temples and through the top. As it grew in, she would continue to soften the base, weaving in other colors for depth and definition. "I might weave in soft auburn on one strand, and a buttery blonde on another, until we get to the point where it is artistically correct, and by that I mean, it goes well with the skin tone, the eyes, even the teeth." Suddenly, the red has evolved into a softer shade of peach, which harmonizes well with the gray, "and this is very flattering to that pale, redhead skin that has changed over the years."

**combination:** Say you're a brunette that has been single-process bleached, possibly with highlights added. Your roots will be salt and pepper. The rest of your hair will be light. The gray will blend in nicely with your blonde, but as your hair grows out, the gray won't be near the blonde. It will exist in a world of dark brunette roots. You've got to uncomplicate things. Beth would begin by making the gray hairs look blonde with a demipermanent color. After taking that down a few notches, she would begin to highlight in two different directions. "Like the way you score a ham," she quips. A trademark technique, known as Color Crossing by Beth Minardi, it leaves less of a line of demarcation. Following this, she would add highlights three times a year, and later twice a year, to maintain a soft, natural-looking gray.

While the overall objectives of softening, blending, and lightening are much the same salon to salon, there are differing ways of achieving them. At the Frédéric Fekkai Salon, color director Constance Hartnett believes in minimal coloring techniques until the gray grows in. "You've got to get it in," she says. "There is no other way." But she can make this a little easier by lightening dark hair to a dusty brown or a dark blonde shade; by muting red until it coexists in a better way with gray; and by adding white and silver highlights to blonde hair, keeping it frosty-looking while the gray comes in.

### Choice 4: You're Just Going to Let the Gray Grow in. Yourself.

Cold turkey is hard for some women. Others seem to breeze right through the grow-in process, reveling in their salt and pepper, loving the changes that seem to happen every day. "Gray hair doesn't sit still," says Amy Trakinski, the lawyer you met in chapter one, who started graying in college. "It seems to have a mind of its own. Sometimes I notice my streaks are more silvery than they were the day before. Some days it looks more washed out."

If you're going to tough it out, you might have to consider yourself a "work in

# positive thinking

"My hairdresser told me,
'People pay a lot of money to get their hair this color.' "
*Deborah Aiges*

"I knew it was growing in nicely; I was getting compliments.
Because I'm in the public eye, I'm identifiable with the gray hair.
I'm not the type of person who would do something to put myself
out there—but since I've got it, I'll keep it!"
*Irene Breslaw Grapel*

"I feel so much better now than when I used to get compliments
on my dyed hair. I used to feel it's not me. But now—it's all me!"
*Setsuko Nagata Ikeda*

"I have great fun with it; people stop me all the time. From the
time I was sixteen, people were telling me how cool it was."
*JoAnne Pinto*

"It's not much of an issue, because I feel young. I am young.
My hair can't take that away from me."
*Dara Roche*

"I just like gray. I've always liked it.
I can't wait until it goes all white."
*Rita Citrin*

"I feel like I'm inventing myself all over again.
It's a new beginning. Hey, this is me."
*Carmine Fuentes*

"I've actually been called foxy with this hair.
And I always say, 'You mean silver foxy.' "
*Joan Kaner*

# going through the change

**Friends, family, and career. Attitude adjustments and emotions.**

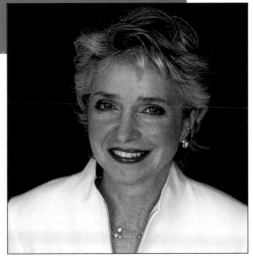

"Hey, Grandma!"

Just what you need.

Penn Curran, of San Francisco, tells the story of a friend of hers. She had made the decision to go gray, weathered the growing-in process, and finally had a very pretty shade of silvery hair that was smartly styled. One day, as she was driving in her car, she did something to irk a rude cab driver. "Hey, Grandma," he yelled out of his open window in protest. That was it, Penn relates. She immediately decided to recolor her hair!

But then she tells the story of another friend, a woman whose husband insists "women who let their hair go gray have a good sense of themselves."

So which is it? What kind of reaction can you expect? Be prepared for both.

You're going through "the Change," and we're not talking about the other one. But it's a little like that. Ten years ago, women never discussed hot flashes, menopausal mood swings, or even perimenopause. Now major cosmetics companies whip up products for "hormonal aging," and aren't afraid to talk about change of life openly. Neither are women. Going gray is the next frontier. It's another change, perhaps the single most important change to your appearance. But many women aren't as prepared for the emotional swings, the personal reassessment, that accompanies graying.

## confidence replacement therapy (crt) For

many years, women felt HRT, hormone replacement therapy, was the answer to the emotional and physical swings of menopause. Is there such a thing for "the change" in your hair color? Whether or not it's accompanied by the creaky bones, the ensuing wrinkles, the shifting of body weight that aging brings with it, CRT is going to make a difference in the way you perceive yourself.

Dr. Anne-Renée Testa, a psychologist who treats self-esteem problems on a daily basis, says women go through a "Gray Alert" during this time. The best thing to do is take action. "Say, 'Honey, it's about time you did something,' then take yourself by the hand and correct whatever is bothering you. And it may not be your hair color."

If you do nothing, it may be insidiously debilitating. Because, like it or not, appearance is tied into self-esteem. "You have to support yourself in a style that you want, then go out and get it," Dr. Testa advises. "Nobody's going to do it for you."

There are women, however, who get stuck in what she calls the "sludge" that is building up in their minds. Women who buckle under a beauty culture that insists perfection is the only answer. This same culture insinuates, "You're old, you're incompetent, you're not sexy, you're invalid, and you are therefore dismissable." Unless you have a core of self-esteem, you begin to believe this. Dr. Testa's CRT advice: Reconnect with your core. Know the value inside of yourself. Know that if you feel good about yourself, and all those things start to happen, you can do something about it. "I tell some women to get the hell out from under themselves," she states. "You can go through your entire life in a little box. You do need someone to give you the courage to get out of it."

Ruth Lawson, at sixty-one, a workshop leader and trainer, knows this feeling too well. With her striking sterling silver braids, she has found both easy-care freedom and a sense of style she likes. But she had to find it herself. "I got tired of going to hairdressers and getting 'old lady hair,' " she says.

> "People have a preconceived notion about what gray hair should look like, or what gray-haired people should wear, or how old they have to be. I didn't even realize I had gray hair until I started noticing their reactions. They had decided who I was. They can put us in a box. I had to break the box."

**getting out** Some women need a box cutter. It may be a friend, someone with whom you are comfortable sharing your innermost thoughts. You need to be able to reach out and say, "I feel life is passing me by. I'm not exercising anymore. I keep choosing the wrong man. I'm being overlooked at work." You need to define whatever is bothering you about yourself. By articulating this, you'll quickly find out if it's your hair color or not.

While a woman may be the best choice for some serious girl talk, even your best friend may not give you an ounce of encouragement to stay gray. And beware your "sisters" at work. So many of the women I've interviewed say women in the workplace are worse than men when it comes to criticizing gray hair. Why is that? I suspected cattiness, but Amy Robinson had a different explanation. "As women, we know what we do to color our hair, all we have to go through—the time, the expense, the itching and the burning. And it's a little threatening to have someone around who doesn't have to go through all of that. It can also be a protective thing. Women know the professional consequences of being gray."

Are comments from women at work really a veiled warning? Or well-intentioned advice? It may be hard to tell. Certainly some will warn of professional dangers lurking down the silver path. But most will couch their comments in terms of aging.

"If anybody said anything at work, it was always the women," says Rita Citrin.

timizing what you are," she says, "instead of trying to look twenty years younger."

## something's different

When things start to click, you're going to get reinforcement from those closest to you, and even from complete strangers. Dr. Testa, who decided stronger lowlights in her hair was what it needed, tells of a maître d' at a restaurant she frequents. "I went in one night, with my new lowlights, and he said, 'You look fabulous.' I said, 'You mean my gray hair?' and he said, 'I don't know about your gray hair, all I know is you look fabulous.'"

We all need nourishment from others, and when we get it, it's "mind blowing," she says. "It confirms what you've done, and in a way, it confirms your own opinion of yourself. Nothing is more valuable."

There will be those who can't quite put their finger on why you look better, but they'll tell you that you do. Or they'll start guessing. Have you had "work" done? Change your hairstyle? Try a new skin treatment? Lose some weight? New man in your life? It can't possibly be your gray hair. Can it? Maybe not. But maybe it *is* what your gray hair prompted you to do.

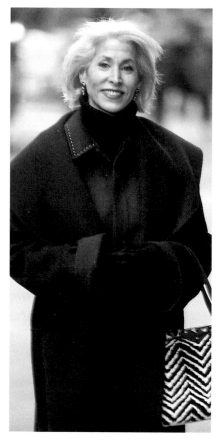

When it all comes together, you'll feel as great as you look! Alice Feder proves it. *Outfit: Lafayette 148 Handbag: Che Che New York*

## the strangest things happen with strangers.

Get ready. Somebody is going to offer you a seat on public transportation. When I asked our panel if anybody had ever experienced this, I was answered with groans, shrieks, and "Yes, and I hate it!" cries of recognition. One woman wailed, "I'm still giving my seat to pregnant ladies!" Another snapped, "I wanted to say, 'You're probably older than I am!'" It happens. Take a deep breath. Find the humor in the situation. And do what you want with the seat.

It could get worse. Deborah Aiges, a youthful-looking woman with hair that's often confused for platinum blonde, tells of bus drivers actually lowering the door steps for her. "I thought he was lowering it for some poor old soul behind me, but I was afraid to look around. And it's happened twice! They see this hair color, and they think you can't get on the bus!"

Gray hair does have its advantages with strangers, however. One very attractive West Coast woman admitted, "I opt to get the senior citizen tickets in our family. Neither of us is old enough, and my husband doesn't look like he qualifies, but with this hair, nobody asks. I get them all the time."

While some women are still burning their AARP cards, others are taking advantage of every kindness, every surprise, that gray hair brings.

Liz Cullumber, the model you met in chapter one, was a speech pathologist who was more than ready for a job change. "My heart was always in something creative, but I didn't know quite what to do with that." At the age of fifty-four, she entered *More* magazine's model search contest, fully confident that her chic gray hair was an asset. It was. She won, netted herself a modeling contract with Wilhelmina, one of the top New York agencies, and now has a booming modeling and TV commercial career. I asked her if gray hair changed her life. Liz thought a moment, then said, "I think my gray hair gave me the *opportunity* to change my life." Perfect point.

Whatever the reaction, startling or flattering, life-changing or simply unsettling, a good attitude is the best response. After all, it *is* just your hair color.

## working through gray hair at work
If there's one unanimous, nagging doubt about gray hair, it's this: Does it work? Literally. Francine Matalon-Degni, the photo stylist you met earlier, tells of a professional encounter of the worst kind: "I'm in an industry where everyone is young and hip, and when I sit across from a photographer who's twenty-eight years old, I wonder, 'Why does he want to hire someone who reminds him of his mother?'" I asked her why, indeed? "He doesn't. He doesn't hire me. Of course I don't know that it's my hair color," she admitted, "but that's how I feel." This is the same woman who loves her hair, who feels she's "earned" the right to wear it any way she chooses.

Security file. More and more companies are doing thorough searches on prospective employees these days, and you will get found out. So if you can't lie about your age, it is pointless to "lie" with the color of your hair. If you're going to camouflage the gray, do it right. Whether you go to a pro, or not, create the most natural effect with a soft, harmonizing color. Allow a few grays to show through, or masquerade as lighter highlights, and keep it real. Anything less artistic creates an obvious subterfuge and will have the adverse effect, calling more attention to your age than a lively, healthy-looking shade of gray.

**a new image starts to emerge** That's you in the mirror. But it *is* a different you, after all. You're looking at someone with gray hair. If you've gone through a gradual process of graying, the evolution that Beth Minardi talks about, your new image isn't going to surprise you. It may take a while to sink in, however. Forty-year-old Amy Trakinski, the lawyer who started to gray in college, had trouble looking at pictures of herself in the few years since she "seriously" grayed. "I would think, Oh, my God, that's me? I really didn't think of myself that way. It would happen when I looked in the mirror every morning, too. But I think I'm past that now," she says.

Okay, it takes a bit of getting used to. If you bleached your hair out to platinum blonde, you'd have to get used to that, too. But look again. There's something else you should see. You should see a woman who has become comfortable with herself, confident about who she is. You should see a woman who has come face to face with the changes that life brings, and who has decided what to do about them. You have reconciled personal fears and other people's opinions, and, most important, you've connected with your own opinion of yourself. Unlike women who go gray by default, you have taken an active role in your appearance. You have considered it from every angle. And you will continue to explore ways to look your best, as you have always done. That's you in the mirror, all right. *Really* you.

| Platitudes | New Attitudes |
|---|---|
| "Hate that gray? Wash it away!" *Clairol advertising slogan for Loving Care, 1960* | "If you hate it, you can get rid of it. But I see more and more women going gray in their own way." *Amy Robinson* |
| "Nobody loves you when you're old and gray." *John Lennon* | "Men love it!" *Dara Roche* |
| "The old gray mare, she ain't what she used to be." *Traditional American folk song* | "I'm more attractive now than I ever was with my natural brunette hair." *Chazz Levi* |
| "Gray is a colour that always seems on the eve of changing to some other colour." *G. K. Chesterton, "The Glory of Gray," 1910* | "I could change it in a heartbeat, if I wanted to. But I don't. And that's my choice." *Alice Feder* |
| "Regrets are the natural property of gray hair." *Charles Dickens,* Martin Chuzzlewit, *1844* | "I like my hair. I've always liked my hair. And if I didn't, I'd do something about it." *Deborah Aiges* |
| "You, my Lady, certainly don't dye your hair to deceive the others, nor even yourself; but only to cheat your own image a little bit before the looking glass." *Luigi Pirandello,* Henry IV, *1922* | "There are some things about yourself that bother you and some things that don't. Gray hair wasn't one of the things that did." *Silvia Maginnis* |

## Platitudes

"Gray hair is a crown of glory."
*Proverbs 16:31*

"There is only one cure for gray hair.
It was invented by a Frenchman.
It is called the guillotine."
P. G. *Wodehouse,* The Old Reliable

"Gray hair is God's graffiti."
*Bill Cosby*

"When your hair has turned to silver,
I will love you just the same."
*Lyrics, Charlie Tobias*
*Music, Peter De Rose*

## New Attitudes

"It's a gift from God. That's my
hairdresser."
*Irene Breslaw Grapel*

"I don't like the expectation that
women will dye their hair."
*Amy Trakinski*

"It's not an accident that women
start to go gray when they finally
figure it all out."
*Licia Hahn*

"My husband thinks it's sexy. He
loves it and always has."
*Francine Matalon-Degni*

# hair apparent

**Just what is gray hair, anyway?
Facts, fiction, physiology.**

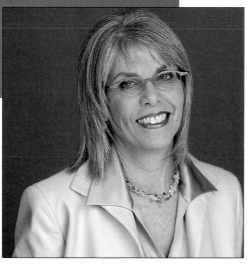

Forget about color for a moment. Let's talk about hair. Why are you going gray? And why now? On average, women seem to hold on to hair color five years longer than their male counterparts. Naturally. (What they do after that is another thing.) The onset of gray is said to start at the age of thirty for males, thirty-five for females. Because various other factors enter into it—like genetics, environment, and health—age is not the single determining factor. It's not uncommon for the process to begin in our twenties (we just don't notice it), and, of course, there are those who start to go gray in their teens.

Why? We can go back to the Greeks again. *Melanos,* their word for "very dark." And *kutos,* for "hollow vessel," the root of "cyte." Put them together, and you have *melanocyte.* Melanocytes are pigment-producing cells—very dark vessels.

Now, not all pigment is very dark. There are actually two kinds of melanin, the pigment produced by the melanocytes. Eumelanin gives the hair its brown to black shades; phaeomelanin, much sparser, reflects as blonde, gold, auburn, and red tones. Hair fiber actually has no color; the cuticle, the outermost protective layer, is transparent. When we see a blonde or a brunette, we perceive color because the pigment shines through. There are, of course, countless variations of shade due to the preponderance of eumelanin or phaeomelanin. Until it disappears.

### when melanin gets the shaft When the cells stop

producing pigment, hair shows an absence of color, appearing gray in contrast to darker shades of hair, or totally white in the absence of other colors; most noticeable when it falls on a nice black sweater.

There's no such thing, really, as "turning" gray. Color doesn't fade away from the shaft; a gray hair comes in gray. It is born without color because the supply of pigment in the hair follicle itself is in short supply. And why? Supply and demand. Let's look at how hair gets its color in the first place.

One of the natural amino acids inside the body, tyrosine, is the raw material of melanin. It is turned into pigment by the enzyme tyrosinase. The more tyrosinase activity, the more pigment is produced in the melanocyte cells.

When the melanocytes are pumping out pigment, it is literally gobbled up by adjoining cells called keratinocytes. You've heard of keratin, hair's chief component. So now, the pigment is visible in the hair, and everybody's happy.

But, somewhere along the way, you start running out of tyrosine. You do not have an infinite supply. And then the enzyme can't make melanin at full capacity. The blood vessels try their best to distribute tyrosine to the bottom of each hair follicle, but when supply is short, there is a loss of color strength. Some follicle depositories have a little more or a little less tyrosine, which means melanin production diminishes at its own rate. This usually occurs in a random pattern at first, starting at your temples and on the top of your head.

In the early stages, the melanocyte cells stick around. They're not very active, but they're there. Later, they decrease in number. So even if you suddenly had your tyrosine supply refilled, you wouldn't have the same number of pigment-producing cells to start cranking out the color again. Eventually, hair appears colorless without any melanin at all.

### a sign of being young. *really* young. This

isn't the first time you've had pigment-free hair. Your first downy postnatal hair, called "vellus hair," was basically uncolored. Don't believe it? Look at the little hairs on your forehead. Vellus hair stays there. It's replaced on other areas of your scalp and body by coarser, pigmented terminal hair. Vellus hair returns to balding heads, but if you aren't losing your hair, the unpigmented hair you see now is good old-fashioned terminal hair. It's not going to fall out at a faster rate than it normally would. It's going to be regenerated time and time again. It's always, from this point on, going to be colorless.

Any little white stray that pops up before the age of twenty in Caucasians, and before the age of thirty in African Americans, can be "officially" called premature. If you were shocked by a gray hair or two at thirty, you may have felt they were premature, but, technically, they were right on schedule. You can, however, find other reasons for what seems to be bad timing. If you want to blame your parents, go ahead. How early we gray *is* determined by our genes, or more specifically, the family code for "turning off" the metabolism of melanocytes. But the genetic connection isn't exactly clear. While early graying may cluster in some families, scientists have not been able to attribute it to a single gene or a common gene. And because there are infinite individual variations, we might as well look to other contributing causes.

**the first frost of aging?** Age may not be the most reliable indicator of when gray hair will appear, but the aging process is the number-one suspect. Common wisdom considers the loss of pigmentation as a sign of "aging normally." But there are so many things that can put your hair on the fast track to aging. We've mentioned the environment, lifestyle choices, and illness. Here's the hit list.

| | |
|---|---|
| Pernicious anemia | Mineral deficiency |
| Thyroid imbalance | Insomnia |
| Free radicals | Depression |
| Menopause | Drugs |
| Stress | Smoking |
| Vitamin deficiency | Vitiligo |

tion, pollution, cigarette smoke and herbicides can spawn free radicals. So does the environment make you gray? In a way.

### vitiligo. a mean streak?
Skin cells and hair cells are so closely co-mingled that when there's a progressive loss of pigment from the epidermis, the hair that grows on that patch of skin will be colorless, as well. This is called vitiligo, a dermatological condition characterized by a depigmentation of skin due to an absence of melanin. Responsible for a streak or swath of gray hair, vitiligo first appears as milky-white patches on the skin. The hair follicles eventually succumb, although they may hold on to their pigment for a while longer. There is a remedy; re-pigment the skin, once the condition stabilizes. If you transplant pigmented skin and hair follicles to the site, the melanocytes in the transplant spread out and repopulate the skin. It may be easier to play up your gray streak for all it's worth.

### scared into being gray?
The notion that a sudden shock can turn hair white overnight has persisted for centuries. It's the stuff of fairy tales and legends, but it won't go away. People actually believe that they have a full head of pigmented hair one day, and the next—poof!—they're stark-raving white. What really has happened is that they have reason to notice the white hair that may have been creeping in all along; it's a visual trick. The shock part comes in because emotional trauma can throw your autoimmune system into a tailspin. This can induce alopecia areata, a genetic autoimmune disorder that causes T cells to mistake hair follicles for a foreign substance. For some strange reason, they attack only pigmented hairs, causing them to fall out. This process may take a few weeks or months, but what's left is the unpigmented hair that was always there. Probably more than the person realized. Suddenly, all they see is white.

But, naturally, stories persist about the exception to the fall-out theory. Ellen Fox, a financial adviser not given to mystical theories, told of her mother's "overnight" graying. Her young brother had fallen out of a second-floor window. He was hurt, but not seriously. The sheer fright of the experience took its toll on her mother's hair, however. The next morning, she awoke with "puffs of gray" scattered throughout her hair. "She didn't turn entirely gray," says Ellen, "but these puffs weren't there when she went to bed."

Setsuko Nagata Ikeda, a violinist who plays with the New York Philharmonic, tells another story. She was in a serious bus accident and was left with a gash in her head. "I was never gray before that, but my hair grew in gray at that spot. For a while I had a streak of white hair, but it all emanated from that spot." The doctors said nothing about it. Setsuko attributes it to the trauma.

If your hair seems to be graying rather rapidly, although you can't claim an overnight sensation, keep in mind the normal process of shedding. Most people lose approximately fifty to a hundred strands of hair a day. The gray strands become more noticeable as the darker strands disappear. A condition called telogen effluvium, in which actively growing hairs suddenly enter telogen, or the resting phase, can speed up shedding to three hundred hairs a day. The cells in the hair's matrix stop dividing, and, as a result, hair begins to fall out, sometimes in clumps. This condition mainly affects women in their forties, fifties, and sixties, as a response to physical or psychological stress. Major surgery, loss of a loved one, depression, or, yes, sudden shock can start the process. So can a shortage of protein or iron in your diet. Back to square one. Your body is in control. And it shifts hairs into resting gear to conserve its nutritional balance. Anorexics, and extreme dieters, beware!

If you can get through life without any of the above affecting you, will you still stop producing melanin in the cortex of your hair? Yes. And is this pigment-free hair any different from your "normal" hair? Yes, again. Although you may not know it. Some women notice no difference at all between the gray hairs and the pigmented hairs on their head. Others will tell you they're coarser, or drier, or frizzier. But, rest assured, even if the hair shows no textural changes, deep down inside, it *has* changed.

## strand and deliver: texture and moisture

A gray hair has a different composition than a nongray hair. Its cuticle is usually thicker. But it is missing its melanin and some of its vital protein. Without melanin, the hair isn't self-protected from the sun's rays, just like skin. And

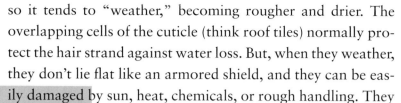

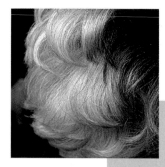

so it tends to "weather," becoming rougher and drier. The overlapping cells of the cuticle (think roof tiles) normally protect the hair strand against water loss. But, when they weather, they don't lie flat like an armored shield, and they can be easily damaged by sun, heat, chemicals, or rough handling. They

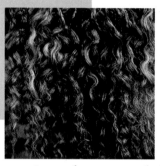

also don't reflect light as well. When cuticle scales are raised, light filters into the hair rather than reflecting off of it. This can account for a dull, lackluster appearance.

Hair texture is a composite of the fiber of the hair and the circumference of the hair. Fine hair has a skinny circumference, and the cuticle is wrapped tightly around the hair. Coarse hair has a fat circumference, and the cuticle is more raised, left ajar. This is the reason why coarse hair gets frizzy, and fine hair, with its tightly compressed cuticle, goes flat. Coarse

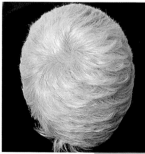

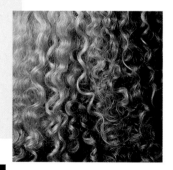

hair may also be wiry and unmalleable, while fine hair will have more shine but no body. So what kind of texture does gray hair have? Any kind it wants. "Gray hair has multiple textures; it isn't always coarse," says Carmine Minardi, co-owner and style director of the Minardi Salon. "It simply fits into one of the twenty-seven different types of hair you can have."

Hair type is determined by texture (fine, medium, coarse); formation (straight, wavy, curly); and amount (sparse, medium, thick). According to a chart developed by Carmine and Beth Minardi, the multiples add up to twenty-seven different possible combinations; there is no separate classification for gray. To find out what type of hair you have, pick a texture, a formation, and an amount. This is your hair category, and it determines the products you choose for shampoos, conditioners, treatments, and styling aids. The next chapter will give you more tips on product selection for nurturing and nourishing gray hair.

**going, going, gone?** Of course, a gray hair is better than no hair at all, but that can happen, too. No, *not* because you're graying. Because you're aging. Half of all women will experience age-related thinning or loss after the age of forty. Because this shows up at about the same time many women go noticeably gray, it's often part and parcel of the gray hair experience, and should be discussed. If you've seen no signs of thinning hair or retreating hairlines, skip this section and *relax!*

Myths aside, you probably won't go bald because you keep plucking gray strands out. Left alone, a single hair has a "life cycle," of four to five years. After that, it falls out and is replaced with a new hair. But sometimes it isn't. Some of the one hundred thousand, plus or minus, hair follicles on your head can simply stop producing new hairs.

If you think a recessive hairline, or baldness, is the result of hair falling out, you are only partially right. The second part of the equation has to come into play. A hair falls out, a new hair doesn't replace it. This can be caused by indolent follicles. Asleep on the job. The hair becomes less dense all over, and the scalp may become visible. It would be wonderful if new follicles would appear, replacing the ones that have gone off duty. But they don't. Your scalp is never going to produce new follicles. You have only the ones you were born with; and this number declines, not increases.

More than 20 million women in the United States alone suffer from some form of "female pattern baldness." Of course, men go through their own "male pattern baldness," but somehow, that's accepted as normal. It is not normal to see a woman going bald. And if it's you, it's horrifying.

**are they going or growing?** Let's go back to the life cycle of the hair shaft to understand what is going on. Hair is not in the same growth phase all over your head. Which is a good thing, or they would all go through the shedding cycle together, and you'd be intermittently bald every three years. Almost 90 percent of the hairs on your head are in the anagen cycle, the growing phase. This lasts about three years. Others are in the catagen phase, just resting, thank you. This is a relatively short period, normally lasting around ten days. And still others are in the shedding phase, the telogen cycle, a period of around a hundred days. Think of this as "molting." Between 50 and 150 strands of hair in the telogen phase will fall out each day. Because these telogen hairs are scattered all over your head, this cyclical hair loss is never noticed, unless you look at your brush.

When the hairs that fall out aren't replaced, and the anagen cycle simply won't kick in, some form of alopecia, the medical term for abnormal hair loss, is at work. Most likely, it is androgenetic alopecia, so called because it is due to the action of male hormones, collectively called androgens. Androgenetic alopecia is the most common cause of female hair loss, the gradual thinning that can begin around the age of forty and increase as you reach menopause. There is a genetic factor at work here as well. You inherit a predisposition for this type of hair loss. And then the hormonal factors kick in. Almost half of all women who experience hair loss can blame it on androgenetic alopecia.

Normally, androgens are present in our bodies in small amounts, produced in the ovaries and adrenal glands. But due to various health factors and medications, the level can increase. High-androgen birth control pills, pregnancy, menopause, thyroid imbalances, anemia, ovarian cysts, and tumors can shift the scales. The level of male androgens does not need to rise to cause a problem; when your female hormones dwindle, the balance of power shifts. To make matters worse, reduced levels of estrogen shorten the anagen, or growing, phase of the hair. So, it's sort of a one-two punch situation. Your growing cycle is shortening, and androgens are gaining control.

### dht: your hair's worst enemy

Back to blaming testosterone. This common androgen converts to DHT, the absolute killer-enemy of the hair shaft. It takes the assistance of an enzyme found in the oil glands of the hair follicle: 5-alpha-reductase type 2, to be exact. Women with androgenetic alopecia have higher levels of this enzyme, especially in hair follicles in the frontal scalp.

As DHT binds to the follicles, it shrinks them until they can no longer survive. The process is called miniaturization, as the blood vessels nourishing the follicle diminish and wither. Death by DHT. No hair can grow where a follicle goes dormant or dies. With this form of hair loss, you will lose hair gradually, but you will not go completely bald. You'll most likely notice diffuse thinning, most likely in the front, temples, and crown. Why the distinctive pattern? Different areas of the head are more sensitive to testosterone and convert it more quickly to DHT.

### can you take a pill or something? Proper
treatment, particularly with antiandrogens and estrogens, can help. Some estrogens produced by the hair follicles actually awaken the follicle from its dormant stage, and tell it to get growing again. Others interfere with the production of the enzyme that transitions testosterone into DHT. But do check first with your doctor; antiandrogens are not recommended for women who intend to get pregnant, and estrogen is not for everybody.

Finasteride (Propecia), originally developed to shrink an enlarged prostate condition, does work, in lower doses, to shrink the production of 5-alpha-reductase type 2, the enzyme that converts testosterone to DHT. But it only works for men; in study after study, it has not been proven to be effective for women. This drug is strictly vetoed for women of childbearing age, because of hormonal effects, and possible birth defects.

### what about a topical treatment? Treatment
with minoxidil, originally a hypertension drug approved in 1988 as a hair-loss treatment for men, and later for women, and minoxidil/tretinoin (Retin-A) combinations have been shown to improve hair growth, increasing the count and thickening the hair fiber. Minoxidil works particularly well for androgenetic alopecia, and is less effective against other types of hair loss. You probably know minoxidil as Rogaine, available over the counter with 2 percent and 5 percent minoxidil.

# it's easy being gray

**Hair care, simplified. The tips, techniques, and products to turn everyday gray into shining silver.**

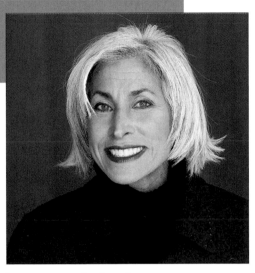

The more I talked to women with gray hair, the more I realized very few did something "special" to keep it in top condition. Many didn't choose a particular shampoo to protect or enhance the color; many didn't use a conditioner; and an amazing number of women didn't even know the names of the products they used on their hair. And yet, their hair seemed radiant, silky, all-out gorgeous. Whatever they were doing, it was working. Could gray hair be the ultimate fuss-free, foolproof hair? Maybe. Or maybe these were just the lucky ones.

The prevailing opinion seemed to be "I've earned the right to have gray hair, and I've earned the right not to be a slave to it." Well, that's good. As long as you like the way it looks. But let me ask you this: Do you take better care of your skin than you did at age twenty-three? That's really all you have to do about your hair.

"Women who say 'I'm not going to do anything' when they turn gray are showing a very natural first reaction," explains Carmine Minardi. "They're responding to the liberation of gray hair, but once they get past that, they want it to be healthier, shinier. Five years down the road, these women want to do something to im-

"People think shampoos and conditioners that are tinted pink or yellow will affect the pure white tone of their hair," says Carmine Minardi, "but actually, this kind of color does not stick to the hair. For instance, look at the Phyto products. There's Phyto Joba, which is yellow, Phyto Rum, which is gold, and Phyto Volume, which is wine-colored. Your hair won't turn these colors."

## "The product color does not affect the color of the hair."

What about shampoos deliberately formulated to enhance color? They may leave a color deposit on your hair, but they don't effectively stain it; the color won't last for more than two or three shampoos.

So, if your gray's got the green meanies, or says hello to yellow more often than you would like, check your water and your plumbing, protect your hair from the sun, reconsider chemical processes, and continue to use a good clarifying or "blue" shampoo every third or fourth time, alternating with a mild shampoo in between. If you use a "blue" shampoo more often than that, your hair very well may end up with a bluish cast! Back to square one.

**easy as one-two-three** Although, admittedly, there are ways gray hair can go wrong, keeping it in good condition can be as simple as you want it to be. Once your hair takes on a glorious gray life of its own, there are really only three things you need to be concerned about.

### 1. Be Sure It's Shining.

Although gray hair isn't a "type" of hair, Carmine Minardi admits it has its own qualities. "The perception of health is harder to achieve," he says. "You have to work at gray hair. And the women who do—those are the ones you point to and say, 'Wow! She looks fabulous.' "

Shine is the most noticeable quality that gives hair the perception of health, and it's important to use the right level of cleansing, the right level of protection, and the right level of after-style products to get it. When light reflection appears to be trapped in the hair, you don't see real detail, and it becomes "one big wad of gray," says Carmine.

**Shine Enhancement** If absolutely nothing seems to give your gray hair the shine and luster you want, there are ways to boost it. Chemical relaxing is one of them. If your hair is strong, in good condition, and not compromised by other chemical processes, chemical relaxing will flatten the cuticle, compressing the fibers closer together. The result: Light reflection is more intense.

Retexturizing the hair is another way to go. It's similar to chemical processing, but it takes it one step further. A heavy flat iron is used on top of the chemical to smooth the cuticle even more, making the hair lie down flatter than ever. "It's the flattest effect, and, consequently, the hair looks even shinier," says Carmine Minardi.

Neither procedure should be tried without an in-depth consultation with your stylist. If your hair isn't up to it, you risk hair breakage.

## 2. Smooth Things Out.

Both husband and wife of the Minardi team believe gray hair is least attractive when it frizzes. "Frizz is old," insists Beth. "Look at anything you love in silver—it's smooth and shiny." That doesn't necessarily mean you have to wear it stick-straight, however. Even wavy or curly hair can have a smooth appearance, if it shows curl definition. "Definition encourages shine," says Carmine, "and that makes the hair appear extremely healthy."

## 3. Select the right products.

At this stage of the game, you know enough to use shampoos formulated for your hair type. You know whether your hair is oily, normal, or dry. But it certainly is the time to escalate into quality treatment brands. They simply have more in the sauce. They're expensive because the ingredients themselves cost more, not to mention the research and development that goes into creating solution-specific formu-

and they do the same thing as silicones. You'll find them in cream-based products like Kiehl's Silk Groom and Kérastase Nutri-Liss.

**give me strength** What if your hair has turned suddenly weaker or thinner? You're going to damage it if you do too much to it, and that includes something as simple as blow-drying. You'll notice a different vitality to your hair if you use products that are formulated to give it some strength and protect it from heat and environmental damage. Better products add fortifiers, like keratin, panthenol, amino acids, and wheat proteins; some add volumizers, like strengthening proteins and polymers for body and control. Polymers are long-chain multiple molecules; they have tensile strength and lend elasticity to hair.

If your hair needs a little moisture, there's moisture and then there's moisture. Any shampoo or treatment that contains water can be said to provide moisture. But you know what happens if you put water on your face and let it evaporate. Your skin gets dry. When you shop for a moisturizing hair product, **look for** ingredients like spirulina, an excellent scalp and hair hydrator (used in top-flight skin moisturizers, too), hyaluronic acid, which binds moisture to the hair, or algae extract, lecithin, bee pollen, jojoba, safflower, or avocado oils. This is healthy moisture, nondrying moisture.

And what about special treatments? Never needed them? Some women equate these with facials and massages, and say they're "not the type" for such indulgences. But there's a reason to give your hair a deep treatment, every now and then, so forget the guilt. This is necessary maintenance. Like it or not, your hair is vulnerable; it's lost its protection. It's out there in the sun and the wind and the rain. And it may be weaker. Be nice to it. It doesn't take long, you can do it yourself, and you don't need to go to a spa.

**look for** protein-based conditioning masks that you can leave in for a few minutes and then wash out. Or, for an intensive shot of care, try a serum treatment. These usually come in pump-activated dispensers, in liquid or lotion form. And they contain higher concentrations of actives, or very targeted ingredients, meant to restore and rehabilitate hair. Simply apply to towel-dried hair and leave in as you style your hair. Three to try: John Barrett's Bee Healed Serum Treatment Conditioning Hair Mask provides intense moisturization; Phytolisse Ultra Shine Smoothing Serum smoothes, shines, and protects hair; and Lancôme Hair Sensation Intense Nutrition Damaged Tips Nutri-Serum repairs and protects dry, brittle ends. You'll be surprised at the way your hair will shine, and you *will* notice a softer, silkier texture.

**a clean future** If you still don't like the ritual of conditioning, fear not. The way we cleanse and condition our hair may be changing soon. "The wave of the future is shampooing, followed by a leave-in cream that moisturizes the hair and becomes a styling aid at the same time," says Carmine Minardi. "This cream is going to have lightweight polymers (bodifiers), so it is really a two in one. You have the cream for detangling, and the polymer to add body. It's all going to be one-shot."

## styling aids: your hair's support system

Somehow the goo, the gels, the mousses for styling have not been abandoned by a majority of the women I talked to. They feel they still need that shape, that hold. Sure, you can borrow your teenager's hair wax, but get to know some products that are formulated for adults. Why? You'll stop over-"fixing" your hair, over-blow-drying it, over-spraying it with drying hairsprays. Your hair will be livelier, shinier, healthier. There are a lot of products on the market that contain kindness with every hold. **look for** hydrating pomades and organic wax creams, beeswax dressings, styling lotions that nourish the hair with vitamins and minerals as they protect it from blow-dry damage. There are texturizing balms and glossing creams, finishing polishes that eliminate frizz while adding shine. Brightening creams and volumizing mousses. The world is your oyster! Investigate!

**the product primer** Need names? Here's a listing of targeted products that aim to restore life, vitality, manageability, and shine to hair. This is a premium list; there may be names and products you've never heard of,

**Bumble and bumble Color Support Styling Lotion—Violet**
*Refreshes color and protects hair from blow-dry damage; nourishes with vitamins and minerals and gives light hold, body, and shine.*

**Sterling Solutions Silver Brightening Hairspray**
*A crystal clear, nonyellowing formula with micro flecks to add extra silvery shine and luster while preventing dulling.*

# Dull, Lifeless Hair

shampoos

**Aveda Brilliant Shampoo**
*Deep cleansing formula to eliminate product buildup and debris.*

**John Barrett C Level Ginger Cider Clarifying Shampoo**
*Provides antioxidant protection; strengthens and fortifies hair while cleansing it of product build up.*

**Frédéric Fekkai Apple Cider Clarifying Shampoo**
*Deeply cleans hair to restore body and shine; eliminates product buildup.*

**Kérastase Bain Satin 2 or 3**
*Nurturing shampoos with gentle cleansing base, to restore shine, smoothness.*

**Lancôme Hair Sensation Intense Nutrition Nourishing Treatment Shampoo**
*Enriched with nourishing and softening ingredients to leave hair clean and supple, with healthy-looking shine.*

**Lancôme Hair Sensation Shine Vitality Gel Shampoo**
*Creamy gel-like formula that combines patented silicone technology and a special polymer to smooth and shine as it washes away excess oils and impurities.*

**Ouidad Clear Shampoo**
*A gentle formula that removes styling product buildup and environmental residue.*

**Sterling Solutions Clarifying Shampoo**
*Brings hair back to its natural state by gently removing normal buildup of shampoos, conditioners, and styling aids; to be used once a week.*

Sterling Solutions Volumizing Shampoo
*With penetrating nourishing vitamins and optical brighteners to bring silvery shine from inside out.*

Sterling Solutions Shampoo and Conditioner
*A one-step treatment that gently cleanses and lusterizes hair with conditioning agents for softness and manageability.*

**conditioners** Aveda Brilliant Damage Control
*Conditions without weight, detangles, and reduces breakage as it adds shine. A prestyling hair spray to protect hair from blow-drying.*

Frédéric Fekkai Apple Cider Clean Conditioner
*Provides sheer conditioning without product buildup.*

Kérastase Nutri-Liss Instant Smoothing Treatment
*Leaves hair soft, shiny; restores discipline and smoothness.*

Kérastase Emulsion Nutri-Instant Enriching Conditioning Mousse
*Detangles and softens without heaviness, smoothing hair fiber and restoring shine and vitality.*

Lancôme Hair Sensation Shine Vitality Express Shine Conditioner
*Light, creamy texture with patent-pending technology to smooth fiber of hair on contact and leave it softer and shinier.*

Ouidad Botanical Boost
*A lightweight, leave-in conditioner that seals in moisture and provides strands with nourishing vitamins and aloe vera.*

Phyto 7 Daily Hydrating Cream
*A creamy, nongreasy formula to maintain optimum moisture levels, replenish and protect. Leaves hair visibly smooth, soft, shiny.*

**treatments** Bumble and bumble Deep Treatment
*Once-a-week nourishment to repair hair, condition, and moisturize.*

Frédéric Fekkai Apple Cider Clearing Rinse
*Removes product buildup and chlorine; leaves hair shiny.*

Kérastase Lumi-Extract Luminizing Cream for Dry Hair
*Supplies shine, softness, and soft hold.*

**Lancôme Hair Sensation Intense Volume Extra Body Conditioner**
*A nonrinse spray-on conditioner that adds volume, body, and shine without weight.*

**treatment**    **Aveda Volumizing Tonic**
*Creates maximum volume and shine with aloe and wheat amino acids.*

**John Barrett Bee Healed Serum Treatment Conditioning Hair Mask**
*Aids in stimulating circulation; intensely moisturizes; helps minimize breakage.*

**Kérastase Expanseur Extra-Corps Fortifying Care for Weakened, Fine Hair**
*Spray-on, leave-in fortifier; improves volume and resistance; helps hold style.*

**Kérastase Ciment Anti-Usure Fortifying Care for Worn-Out Mid-Lengths and Ends**
*Detangles; fortifies from within to add substance, suppleness, and shine.*

**Phytolisse Ultra Shine Smoothing Serum**
*Part treatment, part styling aid; for curls or straight hair; provides smooth finish, shine, and protection without weighing hair down.*

**styling aids**    **Aveda Confixor Conditioning Fixative**
*Combines benefits of conditioner and lightweight styling product; provides medium hold, eliminates flyaways and adds shine.*

**Aveda Phomollient Styling Foam**
*Creates weightless volume; adds shine without buildup or weight; provides light-to-medium hold.*

**Aveda Witch Hazel Light Hold Hair Spray**
*Boosts shine, reduces static, and eliminates flyaways as it provides light hold.*

**John Barrett Bee Big Volumizing Mousse**
*Adds texture, volume, and shine while holding and strengthening hair.*

**Bumble and bumble Thickening Spray**
*Builds body, defines curl, and tames frizz without feeling gummy.*

**Frédéric Fekkai Instant Volume**
*Sprays on to create instant fullness at the roots; protects and strengthens.*

**Kérastaste Volumactive Mousse Bodifying Care for Fine, Flyaway Hair**
*A leave-in styling mousse that strengthens, rebuilds texture, restores shine, and makes hair easier to control.*

**Kérastase Nutri-Body Volumizing Treatment Mousse**
*Adds smoothness, texture, and body; protects hair from blow-dry heat.*

**Lancôme Hair Sensation Intense Volume Extra-Volume Mousse**
*Contains a patented combination of ingredients, including ceramide and special polymers to leave hair soft and manageable, with lasting volume.*

**The Pure Shop Purehair Watercress Finishing Purehold**
*Provides weightless shaping and definition in a natural water-based cream.*

## Frizzy, Unruly Hair

shampoos

**Bumble and bumble Gentle Shampoo**
*Luxurious cream formula; moisturizes and shines as it gently cleanses.*

**Frédéric Fekkai Moisturizing Shampoo with Shea Butter**
*Ultra moisturizing for curly, course, or unruly hair; gently washes and hydrates.*

**Lancôme Hair Sensation Intense Nutrition Nourishing Treatment Shampoo**
*Creamy texture delivers nourishing and softening ingredients to leave hair clean and supple with healthy-looking shine.*

**Ouidad Curl Quencher Shampoo**
*Formulated especially for dry and thirsty curls; pampers and nourishes dry hair with extra moisture.*

**Redken All Soft Shampoo**
*Formulated with an interbond conditioning system of avocado oil, proteins, and amino acids to improve manageability and shine.*

**conditioners**

**Bumble and bumble Leave-In (Rinse-Out) Conditioner**
*Moisturizes hair to tame frizz and flyaways; softens curls without weighing hair down.*

**Frédéric Fekkai Moisturizing Conditioner with Shea Butter**
*Deeply hydrates curly, coarse, or unruly hair; improves manageability and shine.*

**Lancôme Hair Sensation Intense Nutrition Nourishing Daily Conditioner**
*Contains ceramide, silk protein derivatives, and honey to protect and smooth hair surface for maximum shine.*

**Ouidad Botanical Boost**
*A leave-in conditioner to seal in moisture; revives and refreshes curls while it calms frizz.*

**Redken All Soft Conditioner**
*Delivers moisture and softness with avocado oil, proteins to help strengthen, and amino acids for deep conditioning, especially for dry or brittle hair.*

**treatment**

**Frédéric Fekkai Hair Mask with Shea Butter**
*Intensive conditioning treatment that restores moisture and manageability*

**Kérastase Masque Oléo-Relax Relaxing Mask for Dry and Rebellious Hair**
*Nourishes and weights hair, leaving it smooth and shiny, with long-lasting frizz control.*

**Kérastase Serum Oléo-Relax**
*A leave-in that provides volume reduction and discipline, and long-lasting frizz protection.*

**Lancôme Hair Sensation Intense Nutrition Extra Rich Conditioning Mask**
*Strengthens, softens, and smoothes dry, brittle hair with Nutrition System of ceramide and silk protein.*

**Lancôme Hair Sensation Intense Nutrition Damaged Tips Nutri-Serum**
*An ultra-concentrated serum with silicone agents to repair and protect brittle and dry ends.*

**Lancôme Intense Nutrition Smooth and Shine Treatment**
*Lightweight, leave-in formula with smoothing agents to minimize frizz and maximize shine.*

**Ouidad Climate Control Heat & Humidity Gel**
*Protects curls from heat or humidity by absorbing moisture from the air to hydrate each strand and prevent frizz.*

**Ouidad Deep Treatment**
*Nourishes and calms hair; to be used one to two times per month, or as a leave-in conditioner to restore manageability and defeat frizz.*

**Phytodéfrisant Smoothing Serum**
*A leave-in conditioning treatment to rid hair of frizz, improve shine and softness.*

**Phytolisse Ultra Shine Smoothing Serum**
*Part treatment, part styling aid; disciplines unwanted coils and rebellious ringlets to restore a sleek, shiny appearance. Moisturizes and protects without weighing hair down.*

**Redken All Soft Heavy Cream**
*A nutrient-rich treatment for dry or brittle hair, formulated with an interbond conditioning system to restore softness, suppleness, and shine.*

**styling aids**   **Aveda Brilliant Retexturizing Gel**
*Adds medium hold, softness, and shine to coarse hair.*

**Aveda Brilliant Emollient Finishing Gloss**
*Smoothes ends, conditions, shines, and makes hair easy to comb.*

**John Barrett Bee in Control Anti-Frizz Gel**
*Strengthens and conditions hair to add body, with bee pollen to moisturize and shine.*

**John Barrett Bee Hold Style Dressing**
*Lends styling control and shine with beeswax; aids in conditioning hair.*

**John Barrett Smooth Air Styling Spray Gel**
*Contains soy protein to improve condition and appearance of hair; fights humidity.*

**Bumble and bumble Gloss**
*Boosts shine, tames flyaways, prevents static, and creates a light, soft, silky texture.*

**Bumble and bumble Defrizz**
*A light, humidity-proof barrier that calms and smoothes, leaving hair soft and silky.*

**Frédéric Fekkai Straight Away**
*Tames curly hair for styling straight or in frizz-free curls.*

**Frédéric Fekkai Pomade Cristal**
*Provides more shine and stronger hold than a gel for sleek styles.*

**Ouidad Clear Control**
*A hydrating finishing pomade that removes styling product stiffness; helps define and enhance curls.*

**Ouidad Shine Hair Glaze**
*A lightweight serum for thick hair, or blow-drying straight; washes out easily, eliminating buildup.*

**Paul Mitchell Frizz Calmplex**
*Seals hair shaft with natural cornstarch resin for sleek, smooth finish; cuts blow-drying time.*

# Curly Hair

shampoos

**Bumble and bumble Gentle Shampoo**
*Luxurious cream formula moisturizes and shines as it gently cleanses.*

**Frédéric Fekkai Moisturizing Shampoo with Shea Butter**
*Ultra moisturizing for curly, course, or unruly hair; gently washes and hydrates.*

**Lancôme Hair Sensation Intense Nutrition Nourishing Treatment Shampoo**
*Creamy texture delivers nourishing and softening ingredients to leave hair clean and supple with healthy-looking shine.*

**Ouidad Curl Quencher Shampoo**
*Formulated especially for dry and thirsty curls; pampers and nourishes dry hair with extra moisture.*

**conditioners**    Bumble and bumble Super Rich Conditioner
*Detangles, softens, and restores luster to unmanageably curly or coarse hair.*

Frédéric Fekkai Moisturizing Conditioner with Shea Butter
*Deeply hydrates curly, coarse, or unruly hair; improves manageability and shine.*

Lancôme Hair Sensation Intense Nutrition Nourishing Daily Conditioner
*Contains ceramide, silk protein derivatives, and honey to protect and smooth hair surface for maximum shine.*

Ouidad Balancing Rinse
*An oil-, wax-, and fat-free detangler that seals and moisturizers; use as a leave-in conditioner for hard-to-manage curls.*

Ouidad Botanical Boost
*A leave-in conditioner to seal in moisture; revives and refreshes curls while it calms frizz.*

Ouidad Curl Quencher Conditioner
*Formulated especially for dry and thirsty curls; contains extra moisturizers to make hair easier to detangle.*

**treatment**    John Barrett Bee Wavy Curl Enhancing Balm
*Regulates hair moisture to allow curls to look their best.*

Lancôme Intense Nutrition Smooth and Shine Treatment
*Lightweight, leave-in formula with smoothing agents to minimize frizz and maximize shine.*

Ouidad Climate Control Heat & Humidity Gel
*Protects curls from heat or humidity by absorbing moisture from the air to hydrate each strand and prevent frizz.*

Ouidad Deep Treatment
*Nourishes and calms hair; to be used one to two times per month, or as a leave-in conditioner to restore manageability and defeat frizz.*

**styling aids**    Aveda Brilliant Emollient Finishing Gloss
*Smoothes ends, conditions, and boosts shine; makes hair easy to comb.*

**styling aids**

**Bumble and bumble Straight**
*Makes curly hair smooth, sleek, shiny; protects hair from heat styling and humidity.*

**Bumble and bumble Styling Crème**
*Slicks hair, adds body, provides lift at the roots, and defines curls.*

**Frédéric Fekkai Styling Gel**
*Provides firm, natural-looking hold for short or curly hair.*

**Kérastase Elasto-Curl Weightless Curl Defining Mousse**
*Supplies light hold; amplifies curl curve and definition, adding volume and bounce.*

**Kérastase Elasto-Curl Definition Forming Cream for Thick, Curly Hair**
*Provides curl definition, moisturizes, and antifrizz control to leave hair shiny and smooth.*

**Ouidad Clear Control**
*A hydrating finishing pomade that removes styling product stiffness, and helps define and enhance curls.*

**Ouidad Tress F/X**
*A lightweight, alcohol-free styling gel that defines curls without weighing them down; creates an invisible net over curl structure.*

**The Pure Shop Purehair Watercress Finishing Purehold**
*Provides weightless shaping and definition in a natural water-based cream.*

# the product finder

**Advanced Research Labs**
www.advreslab.com

**Aveda**
To find an Aveda store, salon, or spa,
   call 866-823-1425
www.aveda.com

**John Barrett**
John Barrett Salon at
   Bergdorf Goodman
754 Fifth Avenue
New York, NY 10019
212-872-2700
www.johnbarrett.com

**Bumble and bumble**
160 East Fifty-sixth Street
New York, NY 10022
800-7-bumble
212-521-6565
www.bumbleandbumble.com

**Frédéric Fekkai**
15 East Fifty-seventh Street
New York, NY 10022
212-753-9500
444 North Rodeo Drive
Beverly Hills, CA 90210
310-777-8700
www.fredericfekkai.com

**Kérastase**
Exclusive to Kérastase Consultant
   Salons
To find salon near you,
   call 877-748-8357

**Lancôme**
800-LANCOME
www.lancome-usa.com
Select Store Locator to find products
   near you

**L'Oréal**
For ARTec and the Pure Shop
575 Fifth Avenue
New York, NY 10017
www.lorealusa.com

**Paul Mitchell**
www.paulmitchell.com
Select Salon Locator to find salon
   near you

**Ouidad**
846 Seventh Avenue
New York, NY 10019
800-677-4247
www.ouidad.com

**Phyto**
675 Madison Avenue
New York, NY 10021
800-55-PHYTO

**Redken**
212-818-1500
www.redken.com

**Sterling Solutions**
800-327-6151
www.sterlingsolutions.com

# SEVEN

# great style: finding the right image

**Do you really need to change your wardrobe? Or your colors? How to know.**

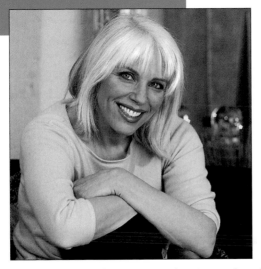

Gray is a neutral. White goes with everything. Silver is elegant. A mix of black and white is always right. When you're talking about clothes, it all makes sense. When you're talking about your hair, suddenly it's a different story.

But it shouldn't be. The same aphorisms that hold true for fashion can apply to your hair color. So what's so hard about getting your clothes and your hair to work together? It all boils down to one thing. You see a different "you" in the mirror.

It is true that you've got a whole new color to contend with. (Forget the non-color, no-pigment thing. When it comes to integrating your hair into a whole fashion look, gray is very much a color!) And that's enough to make you *feel* as if you need to change your wardrobe. After all, your skin looks paler, your face looks different, the colors you used to wear before seem to wash you out even more. It's different than going blonde, women have told me. At least then you have some tone to build color choices around. White or silvered hair gives you no clues. Like a blank slate. Consider this an opportunity.

Licia Hahn, president of a marketing and communications company that counsels on-air television talent, celebrities, politicians, and top-level executives about appearance, looks at it another way. "Color in your hair can actually draw attention away from your face. Think of redheads and blondes. You see their hair, but you spend little time really seeing their face. You see the face in a composite sort of way, but you're not focusing on great features, like beautiful blue eyes or great lips. Women with gray, white, or silver hair have a great opportunity to accentuate their best features."

> ### "Silver is a fantastic background to showcase what God gave you."

To compensate for fading hair color, some women turn first to makeup, amplifying everything. That's not the answer, and we'll deal with that in chapter nine. The second thing they do is to wear all the color they can—bright color; hot color; strong, clear color. Wrong or right?

Hahn, an artist herself, sees gray hair as the frame of a beautiful painting. "Think of the silver frames you have in your house. Do you only put black-and-white pictures in them? Probably not. Or think about a painting you would take to a framer with rich, vibrant colors. You choose a silver frame to make them pop."

**which colors, exactly?** You know that your hair, whatever the color, is the frame for your face. Following Licia Hahn's thinking, it's the frame for your entire wardrobe, as well. Now you have to fill it with color. But which ones? There's more of a consensus on the colors to avoid than the ones to wear, because each woman has to consider her skin tone and her comfort level with the color.

It has to do with your personal palette, as well as the emotional value of the color. If you have a tawny, yellow-based skin tone, for instance, and you've always worn browns and rusts well, you're not suddenly going to look better in certain magentas, reds, and purples. Without a major change in your makeup, intense blue-based shades are just not going to go with your skin. Yes, you'll look brighter, but you could look better. You may want simply to adjust the volume on your palette, making it livelier, or softer (think cinnamon instead of brown, or peach instead of copper; find strength in olive, cinnabar, coral, turquoise), but don't automatically jump to the blue side of the spectrum.

Your eye sees color as either blue-based or yellow-based, whether you are aware of it or not. It's not something you're taught; it's the way the eye works. And, by happy coincidence, Caucasian skin tone is either blue-based (cool) or yellow-based (warm). It gets a little more complicated for women of color. African American skin may be yellow- or blue-based, but it can also have an undertone of red. Asian and Hispanic skin may have more yellow than anything else, but there is a wide range of variation. All very interesting, but how do you use this?

**only important fashion commandment: know thy skin tone!** To keep everything in harmony, you should choose wardrobe shades from color "families" that complement your predominating skin tone. If it's yellow-based, for instance, and you want to wear a shade like pink, go for the sunnier pinks, like geranium, azalea, or coral pink. If it's blue-based, true rose pinks, orchid pinks and magentas are for you. That's how it works, and it's really very simple! *If* you know your skin tone. If you don't, the colors you wear can actually fight with the underlying tone of your skin. Instant clash. You are innately aware of the dissonance, and you are not comfortable in the color.

If you've never been really sure of your skin tone, perhaps now is the best time of all to check with a color expert at your favorite cosmetics counter. As your hair is changing color, your skin tone may not be what you thought it was all along. You'll read more about why this is so when we discuss skin in the next chapter, but for right now, just take this advice: Go find out. You can't develop a wardrobe of the "right" colors without this knowledge.

**feeling color** The emotional value of color is just as important for comfort. Color can have a physical effect on your endocrine system, stirring a response that you simply can't control. It starts from the moment light receptors in the retina of the eye send signals via optic neurons to the visual center of the brain. You see. But the eye isn't the only thing that picks up these signals. The pituitary gland senses them as well, sending out a chemical signal to other endocrine glands in the body.

When the eye sees primary red, for example, the pituitary sends a signal to the adrenal medulla, the part of the adrenal gland that produces epinephrine, otherwise known as adrenaline. Adrenaline is stimulated; it has an arousing effect; you became excited. You feel the color. Other colors, like vivid pink, inspire production of norepinephrine, the chemical that inhibits production of epinephrine, and you have a different response, possibly even an angry one. Marketers have known the psychological and physical implications of color for a long time, and they use them to convince you to buy more, eat more, respond more positively to a product. But you automatically know that certain colors have an effect on you. You feel some clash with your personality, as well as your skin tone, and you're basically right. They're giving you an emotional response you just don't like. On the other hand, you're more comfortable with certain shades because you are physically more comfortable. It gets back to how you feel in a color. If you don't feel right in it, there's a reason.

## from color psychology to fashion No matter

what your inner response is to color, sooner or later you're going to confront an outfit you like, and hesitate about the shade. "A lot of women have a strong opinion of color," says Edward Wilkerson, design director of Lafayette 148. "What they should wear, what they shouldn't wear. Women with nongray hair have the same opinions, so it can't all be about hair color. I observe people all the time—how they dress, what they're wearing—and I find the colors people choose have to do with their profession, everyday lives, and fashion education. And by education I mean the colors they were raised to dress in. They were brought up feeling good in certain colors, and that's what they think they can wear. But none of these opinions should be taken as rules for not wearing color. There should be no rules. Except one—if you don't like yourself in a color, you shouldn't wear it."

> **"I saw a woman with gray hair, wearing a gray sweater and blazing red lipstick. She looked drop-dead beautiful. All I saw was this extraordinary face."**
> *Licia Hahn, president,*
> *Licia Hahn & Co.*

If you've always felt calm and confident with quiet, reticent shades, for instance, you probably don't wear red. It "isn't for you." And that's fine. Gray hair should never be a reason for wearing shades you just don't like. There's no doubt, however, that red gives a great, lively boost to women (okay, *other* women) with gray hair. Since your whole color palette seems to be changing now, maybe it's time to explore. . . .

**ready for red, or not?** The truth about red is that it is many shades. Aside from the revelation that males inherit a preference to look at yellow-based reds, and women inherit a preference for blue-based reds, there are so many variations of red (from orange reds, to berry reds, to brown reds), that it may be possible to find one that doesn't put your adrenals into overdrive. Whatever the tonality, red is a strong favorite for women with gray hair, because it delivers maximum color impact. It's worth experimenting to find the red that works for you.

> **"I notice women with gray hair a lot, especially when they're wearing red, and I think how fabulous they look."**
> *Sandra Wilson, accessories fashion director, Neiman Marcus*

It took Deborah Aiges, the platinum blonde/gray creative director you met in an earlier chapter, some time to find the right red for her. "For a while I couldn't wear red; my skin looked pasty, and my hair looked grayer." She stayed with gray, black, and taupe, added blue, and now has found that a deep maroon red offers her depth and drama without the heightened contrast that turned her skin too white.

> **"My wardrobe is basically black, gray, and beige. But I do have a tomato red sweater, and when I wear it, people say I look great. I think it does kind of brighten me up."**
> *Janice Bryant, copy editor,*
> *Essence magazine*

Francine Matalon-Degni, the photo stylist, did red in reverse. "I used to wear it, but I stopped. It didn't have anything to do with my gray; it was more how I felt inside. It was like drawing attention to myself." She's decided to add a little more color to her wardrobe again, however, so she isn't ruling red out. Look for her in chapter eleven; she's wearing a rich ruby-toned jacket, and looks absolutely fantastic!

**you can't go wrong department** So what colors work, across the board? Black. White. Gray. Navy. Most women have lived with black and white all their lives; they're used to it. And these shades just happen to have the right color energy to coexist with gray hair, providing sharp contrast or a striking complement. Gray is another story. It can provide a wonderful continuity, or it can make a woman feel more blah than ever. ("It blends in too much." "There's too much gray going on.") It takes a little thought to get gray right. But when it works, it's brilliant! And navy gets raves all around, even from women who come to it just because they've gone gray. It's a great foil for pearls, another face brightener. And it's a super confidence booster; navy is one of those "power colors" that is appropriate at most times.

Betty Halbreich, the wardrobe maven from Bergdorf Goodman's Solutions department, whom you met in chapter four, counts sophisticated, successful women, film studio execs, and television stars among her clients. She never minces words when she's working one on one, and she offers the same smart advice in her book, *Secrets of a Fashion Therapist*. Halbreich happily revealed a few more secrets about the "right" colors for gray to me. "My instinct with gray hair is the pinks, the sapphire blues. But designers aren't giving you sapphire blue. They don't have a clue what you're talking about. It's not like laying out paint chips, the way women used to do when they "had their colors done." You can lay out all these pretty colors, but designers don't give women pretty colors to wear. And that's why black became the safety harbor. I'm so sick of black. Most of the women I see are, too. They want to get away from it."

Halbreich finds it's "so easy to dress" women with gray hair. "You can put them in gray, in colors. White is good if it's that sharp white—chic white. And satins are good; they have some glow to them. You have to stay away from beige, but that's about the only thing. And we're living in a beige world right now." But then she goes right back to gray. "I saw a woman with grayish blackish hair the other day, in all tones of gray, head to foot. She looked great."

**the case for gray** Women who know the power of gray know that it lies in the textural mix. It's true, you've got to get some contrast going, but you can do that with a blending of textures, or with the instant light of metals and shine. Pair a soft gray mélange sweater with a slick gray leather skirt or pants. Swirl it all up with a tweedy, salt-and-pepper shawl, and you've got the textural mix that brings gray to life. Metallics add polish to any look, and you don't have to save them for night if you combine them in shine-and-matte ways. The variations with texture are endless: Wear a silvery satin camisole under a deeper gray pinstripe suit. Team a matte-gray knit top with shining, silvery shantung pants for evening. Add the hard shine of a "silver" metal chain belt to a soft gray sweater dress. It's the contrast that counts: Think light with dark, matte with shine, soft with slick—and you've got it.

Playing gray all the way, in a single texture, gives a modern, minimal look. And that's when you can add something else—a light, lifting color, something bright white, or an unusually intriguing accessory. Try a chunky cuff bracelet with nuggets of stones, or a carved oriental pendant with a silken tassel—something that draws the eye. It's the ideal screen on which to project any mood, any style, you want.

Psychologically, gray has a stronger impact than you might think. Licia Hahn reminds us to "look at the things we are surrounded by; the buildings, bridges, structures of great strength, durability, and power. Subliminally, we associate gray with strength, with things that support us and hold us up. Gray is a metaphor for the strength women see in themselves."

If you've stayed away from gray before, think of it as a transition color, midway between black and white. "If you've been wearing black, black, black, gray is a great color to graduate to," says Hahn. "Black is not as forgiving." She believes that gray is every bit as flexible as black, a color that can go from day to evening.

"There's an uncomplicated purity to gray," she says. It's about a certain state of mind. Gray can be both quiet and dramatic. This is a very powerful look. It's a way to make a statement and to express individuality. Women with gray hair have this wonderful luminescence, and dressing in gray plays it up perfectly."

**color it wrong** There are colors that women with gray hair think twice about. It's not the fashion police who are saying this. It's the women who have been there, done that, and didn't like the following shades at all:

**beige** is the number-one color women with gray hair feel they absolutely cannot wear. And all colors related to beige: **ivory, cream, vanilla, off-white, ecru,** even **camel.** One woman I spoke to was "dying" to purchase a camel coat, but she wanted some advice. When I suggested she team it with a pink or red scarf, her face brightened. That's the point—put something brighter, softer, or prettier close to your face, and it will work. Forget beige or off-white (which can have much the same effect as yellowing in the hair), and go for crisp white. Sharpen the shade, and you go from blah to bravo!

**brown** is a split decision. Women with pure white hair prefer black, if they're going to wear a dark shade, for a stronger contrast. Women with salt-and-pepper hair tend to feel that brown isn't entirely complementary. But if there is enough "pepper" in the hair to support it, a deep, rich brown, or a brown lit with white, can be terrific. When I interviewed Joan Kaner, the salt-and-pepper senior vice president and fashion director of Neiman Marcus, she was wearing a brown pin-striped suit and looking very smart. "I fall in love with a color, so I buy it," she says. "I never think about what color my hair is."

**acid or lime-based greens** are colors that give some women with gray hair difficulty. Yet those with tawnier complexions do well with these shades, especially in the summer, if they bronze. Those who don't tan, and women with cool skin tones, find greens with a little blue added more wearable; the pine greens, the teals, the aquamarine tones. They're softer against a pale complexion, but they work to add brightness.

**yellow** doesn't win many votes. "Few women look great in yellow," says Licia Hahn. "But it isn't your hair that's doing it. It's just a hard color next to most skin tones." If you can get away with it, it's an instant brightener. Yellow is the "fastest" color for the eye to see, and so it is the first color you notice. It calls attention to itself immediately: To make it compatible with a complexion framed in white or silver, Hahn advises warming up the color in your face first. "There are a lot of things you can do; the self-tanners are great," she says.

Licia Hahn feels the color "formulas" that women latched on to several years ago don't apply today. "That spring/winter color thing was fine for a while, because it got women thinking about color in relation to themselves, but it tends to put women in color boxes. I think women have more imagination."

### a wardrobe strategy

If you use your new hair "color" as an excuse to buy a whole new wardrobe, it's just that. An excuse. Because it isn't really necessary. You might find a new piece or two will work wonders. Start by pitching what doesn't look good on you at all anymore. Save the basic shades like gray, white, black, navy. Keep the clear colors that work. Then find a base to build on.

Joan Kaner, the fashion director of Neiman Marcus, suggests that you start with darks or neutrals. Black is a great all-day, all-night transitional color, or you may choose a silvery/gray neutral or a taupe/brown neutral as your base, depending on your skin tone. And then freshen it with a color piece.

"Each season, I always buy black tops and black pants," she says, "and then I add a jacket in various colors—burnt orange, violet, a frosted or grayed pastel. That way, I'm bringing color to my face. It's very hard to wear color head to toe. It's much better to keep color as an accent top piece over a neutral base. It applies instant benefits where they can do the most good."

While a base gives your wardrobe strength, pastels can add just the right amount of softness. But not wishy-washy pastels, Kaner advises. "I'm talking about ones that have a little more character; celadon, sea foam, or old rose. They have a

> "I love brights, and I do well with colors, but I don't buy things for my hair. I buy things for me. I shop for the kinds of things that appeal to my eye and that I look and feel good in."
> **Ruth Lawson, workshop leader and trainer**

little gray added, and that looks very good with gray hair. Yes, you can wear pastels, but they have to have something to them, a little bit of a bite."

## new image, new you? No matter what your age when

you start to gray, it has the effect of making you feel older. Maybe it causes your confidence to slip a notch. Is it time to go trendy, dress younger? No on both counts. And double no to dressing like your daughter. It's silly, and it isn't practical. Especially if you're updating your wardrobe.

Betty Halbreich advises women to get the sequence of change right. "First, you've got to work on the hair, then the makeup, then you come down to the clothes. But a woman does not let her hair go gray without a good feeling about herself. She shouldn't have to go trendy. She can revitalize with color, or a new look, but how about looking sophisticated? You are either dressing like a kid, or in real-people clothes, there's just nothing in between these days. Yes, you're going to want a new look, but that doesn't equate with a young look," she says.

"You shouldn't be buying trends," agrees Joan Kaner. "It's better to build on your wardrobe. Buy nothing that's going to be obsolete in six months. Clothes today are too expensive, and nobody should have to get rid of an item in six months."

Designer Edward Wilkerson doesn't recommend a drastic change. "If you have style, if you're accustomed to looking a certain way, the best thing is to maintain that style. What you should do is integrate [gray hair] into your style. Work with it, and keep it looking as great as possible, but keep doing what you're doing in terms of dressing."

## little tricks, big difference There are, of course,

ways to update your wardrobe and give your style—your *own* style—a more modern look. "I don't ever think a woman should go trendy as she ages; I feel very strongly about that," says Licia Hahn. "But that doesn't mean you can't be creative. And you can do this in subtle little ways." Her advice is to be more playful, to acknowledge your personality, and your best assets. "If you've always worn a jacket, get rid of it once in a while. Try a pretty blouse. Show off your waistline if it's good.

Show off your legs with the flip of a ruffled hem, pleats, or little slits. Wear a scooped-out neckline to show off a good décolletage."

> "Celebrate your sexuality because it's not over until it's over."

"I always get a good sense of how far I can go with a client," Hahn continues, "but then I tell her to push it a little bit. Dare to step out a little further. It's about re-defining yourself, but still being true to yourself. Find your best feature and then have more fun with it. Integrate classics with something joyful—I call it classic with a twist, with your eyebrow raised a little bit. Don't take yourself too seriously, and do enjoy who you really are."

## never underestimate the power of accessories

Clothes can't do it all. That extra bit of brightening your skin might need can come from accessories. That pretty touch of color near the face can be a necklace or an earring. And something that makes a statement might be a last-minute add-on, rather than an outfit. Accessories, once thought of as unessential luxuries, are real workhorses for the modern woman. They say more about her personal style than anything else.

"The way you dress is the way you express yourself; it's your handwriting," says Sandra Wilson, accessories fashion director of Neiman Marcus. "But accessories are your signature. You can always find something special, something a little distinctive, that revitalizes your wardrobe."

Accessories are personal items; they can't be prescribed for every woman. Proportion, coloring, and comfort levels enter into the picture. Shawls, for instance, have been around for a long time, and they're great for adding a touch of color and drama. "But a woman should only wear them if she is dramatic," says Wilson. "She'll be able to carry it off better than someone who is always going to fuss with it. If a shawl-savvy woman needs a color boost, this is how she'll get it."

Sandra Wilson does caution women on the use of scarves, however. Those square, silk status scarves "can be very old." It's better to put something soft next to your skin, like a great texture, or even fur. "Silver fox looks fabulous with gray hair," she says, used in place of a scarf at the neckline. When you think you have to add color to a dress, or a suit jacket, texture might just be the way to go.

### the spotlight of light
Accessories give you the chance to add dazzle and impact where you need it most. "In general, if a woman feels she is paling in certain colors, she can turn to something that has some importance," Wilson advises. "For a long time, we were in a phase of minimal jewelry, but now large, somewhat organic, semiprecious stones look good. Natural stones like agates and rutilated quartz, or precious, faceted stones come in such wonderful colors for gray hair: the citrines, tourmalines, and peridots. They add an amazing light, especially around the face. Gemstones are like a cosmetic, the light going through them gives you an emotional uplift; they're a cosmetic to the face and the soul."

Pearls are born to add light, as well. So are metals. Platinum, silver, gold. Wait a minute—*gold?* Some women, as they gray, opt for silver exclusively, ditching gold like it's the basest of all metals. Of course, silver is quite complementary to gray and silver hair; that's a no-brainer. It also lends a special coolness to black, white, and many other colors you wear. But don't think you have to abandon gold. Gold has a gleam of its own, and it isn't going to "clash" with your hair. It's simply going to be gold. Metals and stones carry their own optical value, and they never, ever need to blend in. If you're still a bit wary of it, Sandra Wilson advises you to look for rose gold, adding a nuance of color that takes it a little further away from yellow. "Rose gold is very pretty, very special," she says, "and it's particularly nice with gray hair."

### the little arrow effect
Accessories are like computer arrows; they direct the eye to the immediate area. What better way to highlight your best features. "If you have great hands, show them off with bracelets. If you

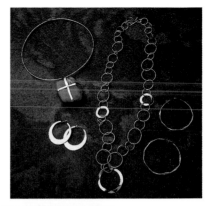

have nicely shaped ears, wear more attention-getting earrings," says Licia Hahn. "You're adding interest to complete what is there." Of course, the reverse applies. "If your neck has those horizontal lines in it, or your chin line is sagging, don't think you're going to hide this behind a necklace. You're not. You're going to drive the eye right to it."

Remember Barbara Bush and her triple-strand pearl necklace? It added light to her face and a great signature look to her style, but we all knew what she was doing. Reminiscent of the elegant deception practiced by women of a certain age (and era), who would wear high-rising, multiple-strand chokers, the "dowager's necklace" today is another name for those rings of wrinkles around the neck.

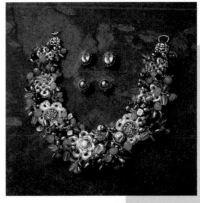

A more modern subterfuge for a lined neck is a scarf or a higher collar, but styles continue to change. "I'm finding nobody wants to wear turtlenecks anymore," notes Betty Halbreich. "So I bead them up. Lots of colored beads." Back to Barbara. But this time around, beads are carved, and strung in intriguing combinations. They can be shaped like objects from nature, like a shell or a leaf. They can be a mix of metals and stones and pastel-colored pearls. They can be clipped with a pendant or drop. And they can twine and twirl around one another, compounding the interest of each strand. The point is, there's a lot going on that's so intriguing, they're more than mere camouflage.

The point is to know what you're getting in a shorter necklace, and what you're not. See what it offers you. If it's color and light and a pretty glow to the complexion, it's

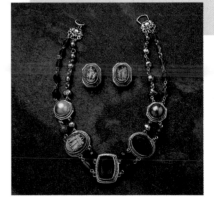

Going beyond gold and silver. Mix metals with gleaming, carved, and colored stones or small beads. It's a way of adding light and intrigue. Items shown here are from Stephen Dweck and Ippolita.

**113**

going to do something for your hair. If it's just going to sit there, dull and flat against your skin, a long, dramatic pendant might send the eye to a better place.

**having an accessories "style"** Accessories can become a uniform, a code to your dressing. You may always wear certain pieces because they feel good, or you're comfortable with them, or they have special significance. This, too, becomes a signature, and there's nothing wrong with that.

"It's all about what you feel inside. Whatever the trend is, you can adapt it, experiment with something you never thought you could wear. But you don't have to go with the flow," advises Sandra Wilson. "Some women love dangle earrings; others love large earrings. Smaller, more intricate shapes are in style at the moment, but all that means is you might scale down a bit without giving up on the shapes and the styles that you like."

> "You have to maintain your personality. But you do go through cycles, so this gives you some leeway. Don't get stuck in a rut."

A definitive style may also have to do with wearing memorable pieces. When Licia Hahn advises her clients about accessories, she endorses the idea of pieces that make an impact. "Don't wear a bracelet unless it is a great bracelet. And by that, I don't necessarily mean more expensive, or even real jewels. I mean a bracelet that has a sense of importance, scale, architecture."

**building blocks: the zone approach** With her artist's sensibility, Hahn thinks in terms of adding blocks of color, "like Mondrian," she says. "Think of your body divided into zones. One zone stops at the shoulders, another zone goes down through the hips, and the third zone is your legs. Don't complicate all these levels with busy-ness. If it means matching your panty hose to your shoes, and to your pants or skirt, you're giving yourself a solid zone, and an elegant, fluid line. There's nothing jarring about your look."

Another way to uncomplicate a look is to think about the hidden accessories in your clothes. Your jacket may have lapels that carve out a certain line. Or it may have interesting clasps that add an element of jewelry. "That's all you need," she says, "to use a technical fashion term, don't gook it up."

**the pleasure principle** The point of accessories is to bring focus to what you're wearing. To add a bit of dash, a touch of surprise. To break up a color that may not be good next to your face, your hair. To add texture or polish. That's what accessories are there for. And to do one other important thing—to delight.

# EIGHT

# great skin: beating the blahs

**Is your face turning gray, too? How to deal with dullness, washout, loss of glow.**

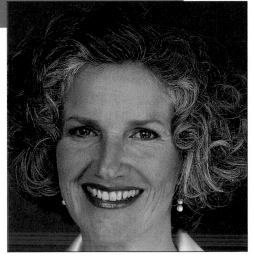

You look at your face, and it's a whole new ball game. Without its surrounding frame of color, your skin tone looks paler, your complexion looks duller. There's some sort of vibrancy that's missing. There are a multitude of reasons, of course, most of them connected to the normal aging process of skin. You can run, but you can't hide; and you certainly can't hide what's happening to your complexion under a bunch of makeup. Get the skin right first. Find a regime to revitalize, optimize, and repair, and then you can use cosmetics sparingly, or dramatically, as you prefer.

Even if your hair loses pigment at a young age, you may notice a paler, grayed-out look to your skin. Why? To begin with, color has been erased from your face. The color from inside your hair shaft. Remember your pigment facts: Color is actually in the cortex of the hair; we perceive color because the pigment shines through. This reflective quality affects your skin tone as well. And it isn't always a good thing. Dark-colored hair can play up the shadows in your face, causing you to appear older. Light-colored hair can hype the yellow tone in your skin, and you can look more sallow. But no-color hair shows the real you; the real skin tone color. You may not have seen it before; you may not like it now. Suddenly, you're paler, ruddier, more sallow, or, yes, even grayer and ashier than you ever knew.

### where did the glow go? The number-one gray hair complaint: My face looks dull, dull, dull. This can happen no matter what age your hair turns gray. It can also happen if you don't turn gray. It's not your hair. It's your skin. Suddenly you've lost that "radiance" beauty companies talk so much about. There's just no glow.

Kathy Dwyer, the founder and CEO of Skinklinic in Manhattan, and former president of Revlon USA, has a way of demystifying what happens to skin as it ages: "Skin is originally meant to absorb insults and injury to your body, so your internal organs are protected. That's what it's there for. It takes the bullet. So, damage is done, over time."

The aging of skin is a gradual process. It can start prematurely, with damage inflicted by UV rays, free radicals, and environmental pollution. And it can accelerate when a woman's hormone supply is depleted. Menopause accounts for the most rapid changes in the skin, causing it to appear lifeless, older, drier, with alarming speed. Dry skin is like dust; it can't reflect anything. Your skin loses its youthful glow, as well as its firmness and vitality.

### a dead cell is a dull cell As a cell goes through its life cycle, it makes its way to the surface of the skin. But dying cells get lazy; they cling to the skin. When that happens, your complexion looks as dead as the cells. The surface of your face can appear ashen or pasty. Worse yet, edges of withered cells tend to curl up, like a leaf, so the skin no longer has a smooth, reflective surface. It looks duller and feels rougher.

"The rate of cell turnover changes," says Kathy Dwyer. "When you're sixteen, it's every twenty-eight days. Dead skin cells just don't hang around on young skin. So there's always a fresh, new skin on the surface. When you're forty, it takes anywhere between thirty-eight to forty-eight days. As you age, this fresh new skin doesn't appear that often, and you begin to notice some sort of loss of vitality. Your skin doesn't glow."

Shedding is the way skin renews itself. As a cell nears the end of its life cycle, it releases lipids (fats) and proteins, two of the chief structural components of living cells. The lipids hold water in the skin. But as the uppermost layer of skin, the stratum corneum, thins with aging, this lipid supply decreases. The natural barrier function breaks down, moisture levels are no longer maintained, and the skin becomes drier and more vulnerable to environmental damage.

That's when all sorts of things can go wrong. For one, elastase, a natural enzyme, is released in response to environmental stress; and while its normal function is to break down old elastic fibers, sun exposure can cause it to become overactive, causing a significant change in the elasticity of the skin. Read sagging and wrinkles. Elastase can damage both tone and texture, resulting in a pebbly surface feel. Pebbly isn't radiant.

## what about the wash-out? The second most common complaint that comes along with gray hair is that skin looks washed out, paler. If you're in your twenties or thirties, absence of color in your hair has a cooling effect on your complexion. Think what happens when you wear a charcoal suit. You want to brighten it, in some way, with gleaming accessories or a pretty-colored top underneath. When it's your hair that's charcoal, you want to brighten your face.

It's true, skin tone does fade through the decades, but there's something else going on. For women in their forties and beyond, the fade-out effect may have more to do with a natural thinning of skin. It loses density; the cushiony little layers flatten out, and the skin becomes a little less opaque. A thinner skin reveals veins and shadows that weren't noticeable when you were younger. You may think your skin looks a bit paler, a bit grayer, when it's really only more transparent.

There's another reason skin can look paler; it's less defined by curves and highlights. "It's not the color of your skin that's necessarily fading," says Dwyer. "You start to lose collagen or body fat. So you go flat under the eyes, where it used to be so puffy your mascara would smudge, flat around the mouth, flat around the lip line. It's that flatness you're picking up on."

are doing in biotechnology today is to protect and preserve the natural function of the skin. When skin is functioning like it should, it is healthy strong, and youthful-looking."

Underneath all the puffery of advertising, all the pretty model faces, all the claims for "radiant, younger-looking skin," there is science at work. There are a few tricks, as well, and we'll get to them later. But for right now, you can take care of your skin in the best possible way—you can bring back the glow and fight the fade-out—by taking advantage of the new products on the market, and following a simple three-part strategy:

## All you need to do is bump, dump, and plump.

# 1. bump Off with the old. When you stimulate the natural
shedding process of cells, you'll lose the dry, dead ones that cling to the surface of the skin. Exfoliation has been with us since washcloths and loofahs, but there are far kinder ways to treat the skin of your face. Aha. Enter AHAs, alpha hydroxy acids. Derived from natural fruit and milk sugars, they've been improving skin since Cleopatra's sour milk baths, but it was dermatologists who began using them seriously. In 1990, the Estée Lauder Company was the first to bring AHA's to the department store counter, in Origins' Starting Over, and, later, in Fruition. Then, suddenly, they were everywhere—in moisturizers and night creams, in cleansers and body lotions. But it *was* possible to get too much of a good thing. As products were introduced with ever-increasing levels of these "natural fruit acids," high percentages of alpha hydroxy proved to be irritating to the skin.

Estée Lauder turned to glucosamine, an ingredient that lessens cell adhesion, to achieve the same results without irritation; other companies switched to oil-soluble beta hydroxy acids (BHAs); still others combined alpha with beta, promising gentler exfoliation. Skincare had turned into alphabet soup.

### A Kinder, Gentler Alpha

Exfoliation is still the best way to get the glow going. If you tried an alpha hydroxy product long ago, and it irritated your skin, things have changed. Can they still irritate your skin? Yes. They also increase sun sensitivity, so you must use a sunscreen with both UVA and UVB protection. That said, today's alpha hydroxy products follow FDA guidelines to reduce side effects. Now most consumer products contain an AHA concentration of 5 to 8 percent and a less acidic pH of 3.5 to 4. Trained cosmetologists can use a 20 to 30 percent concentration, and dermatologists, 50 to 70 percent. So that gives you an idea how mild the products you can buy really are.

Or you might try a product that has a beta, or a beta/alpha combination. How will you know which is which? Common "alphas" listed in ingredients include lactic (milk), glycolic (sugar cane), and tartaric (grape) acids. You might also find "triple fruit acid" or "tri-alpha hydroxy fruit acids" or "alpha hydroxy and botanical complex."

If you're looking for a beta hydroxy, look for salicylic acid, tropic acid, trethocanic acid. An alpha-beta mix is indicated with malic (apples and pears) or citric (oranges and lemons) acids. Or it simply might say "a blending of alpha and beta hydroxy acids." If you want to skip the acids altogether, try a product containing a different type of exfoliator, like glucosamine. Experiment, learn, and find out as much as you can. It's worth the time to find an effective cell shedder that your skin can tolerate.

You don't have to buy a special kind of product because these ingredients can be found in the kinds of things you use in your daily skincare regime. **look for** exfoliating ingredients in daily cleansers, moisturizers, night creams, and foundations. But do go gently. Everything you put on your face shouldn't contain exfoliators. If you start with a moisturizer that bumps away cells, you may need nothing more. Or you may combine an exfoliating cleanser and once-a-week special treatment. "It's better to work at getting the glow back in a combination of ways," says Janet Carlson Freed. "It's kind of like the way we should eat—everything in moderation. You'll know if your skin feels overtaxed."

**full-service** When you supplement the products you use at home with professional treatments, it maximizes the results. "Treatment is the primary way to bring back the glow; you can't get the same level of change without it," says Kathy Dwyer. "Products you buy off the shelves don't contain the same levels "glue," the desmosomes, that holds the cells together. Because salicylic peels cut through skin lipids and oiliness, however, they can be drying; they are most useful for oily or acne-prone skin, or to break down blackheads and whiteheads.

Glycolics are the treatment of choice for normal, dull, or aging skin. "Glycolic-based peels increase cell turnover," says Ellen Lange, president and founder of Ellen Lange Skin Science, "and this improves the texture and look of skin."

After a series of glycolics, however, there can be a desensitizing effect. Some women claim they stop working altogether because "there's nothing left to peel." The truth is, there are always dead cells rising to the surface. But skin can thin if you eliminate faster than you replenish. Glycolic peels come in a variety of strengths. At Skinklinic, for example, 20 to 50 percent is considered light, and 50 to 70 percent medium (the 70 percent is buffered, to lower irritation). But wherever you have the peel performed, know the strength you're getting. You can proceed up the scale gradually, or stay in the lower ranges. According to the estheticians at Ellen Lange, "A lighter-strength peel allows you to do it on a regular basis, and you will have effective results."

## one from column a, one from column b?

Should you just have a facial and be done with it? Or maybe a microdermabrasion treatment once a year? Well, like a jolt of caffeine in the morning, any treatment will jump-start your skin. But it's not going to keep it performing. "You need to do more things as you go forward," Skinklinic's Kathy Dwyer advises. "Sometimes you can alternate between two treatments, or sometimes do a combination. But don't have downtime, especially after the age of thirty-five. The more you do, the more your skin thinks it has to do. That takes a while. What you *will* notice, immediately, is brighter skin. It will have more clarity. And it won't have that dullness."

If all of this sounds a bit excessive, take a look at your skin without makeup. In a bright light. Wouldn't go out this way? Dwyer, who admits to doing a bit of everything at age fifty-four, was wearing no makeup at all when we talked. Her skin tone was even, her complexion was pearly pink—there wasn't a line or a wrinkle in sight. And she *glowed*.

**self-service** If you don't have the time, the money, or the inclination to go after a slew of professional treatments, there are many things you can do to get the glow going at home. Even if you regularly have professional treatments, you don't get a free pass in the home-care department. It's what you do every day that accelerates and maintains what the pros have done.

Dr. Dennis Gross, New York dermatologist and founder of MD Skincare, likes to equate skin care to fitness: "Skin is like a muscle, it does better by working out a little bit every day. The skin likes the fact that it's being worked upon and improved upon in small increments. It's day-to-day treatment that gives the skin its best results.

"If a woman is going to take the time to work on her skin, she should be doing things that give her immediate and long-term benefits, and by that I mean addressing the underlying difficulties in the skin and rebuilding the structure," Dr. Lydia Evans advises. Good skincare can start at the most fundamental level, according to the doctor's prescription: (1) Use a good cleanser. (2) Use a good moisturizer. (3) Protect skin from the sun. From there, Dr. Evans recommends a series of peels complemented by regular use of products containing gentle exfoliators.

There are many products for do-it-yourself glow power. Once the domain of dermatologist and boutique brands, skin resurfacers are now cropping up among the big names; the brands you can buy in department stores and drugstores. Look to the Shopbox for some of the best bumpers around.

## shopbox

• **Prescriptives Dermapolish** is a three-part system developed to provide "professional" results at home. Includes a Treatment Cream, containing microcrystals combined with soy proteins and aloe vera; a Post Treatment Soothing Mist of Brazilian red algae extract, green tea, and aloe vera; and a Lipid Barrier Cream of shea butter, soybean protein, and antioxidants to rehydrate skin.

• **Ellen Lange Retexturizing Peel Kit** is a four-step process, including a peel prep, peel accelerator, peel solution, and postpeel cream, designed to speed up the skin's natural exfoliation. The peeling solution is a blend of glycolic acid, special enzymes, and microbeads that foams, tingles, and absorbs into the skin. This is to be followed by the cream, to soften and hydrate the face.

*(continued on next page)*

• **MD Skincare Alpha Beta Daily Face Peel** uses two hydroxy acids, alpha and beta, for gentle peeling. It is a two-step process; the at-home "kit" contains two separate types of active-infused pads. "You have to deliver the right ingredients in the right way," Dr. Dennis Gross says. "This two-step peel works to rid the skin of dulling cells with the first pad, and then the second pad brings green tea and vitamin C to the skin to give it a calmness and a finish that makes it look wonderful. It's effective because you can use it every day."

• **Georgette Klinger AHA Skin Refining Surface Exfoliator** is a dual-action, wash-off product that gives you both immediate and continual benefits. Gentle sloughing beads polish skin's surface for instant smoothness, while the alpha hydroxy acids work long-term. For face and body.

Okay, got the face glowing? Look down. How about your décolleté? Your shoulders and arms. Your elbows, knees, and hands. These can do with a little bumping, too. Body skin is a bit thicker, but it can benefit from cell turnover as well, and there's no sense in having a glowing face and a dry, flaky body.

L'Oréal's Body Expertise line is a good one to turn to, providing total body care in a number of ways. To start shedding the deadheads, there's Exfotonic New Skin Revealing Exfoliator, a creamy, glycerin-based product, that contains both alpha hydroxy acid and microbeads. Use it two to three times a week to restore smoothness and even skin tone. For daily body moisturizing, there's NutriFit Intensive Firming and Moisturizing Lotion for Body & Hand in two formulas, one for dry and one for extra-dry skin, so you can vary the remedy to the condition of your skin or the seasons. If your body skin is bone dry, the extra-dry formula supplies a ceramide and shea butter complex to help replenish the skin's lost lipids. Now you can glow down to your toes!

## 2. dump

If your skin isn't responding to what you've always used, it may be time to dump the old stand-bys. Skin gets tired of the same-old, same-old too, so new products can actually jump-start it. And the newer biotechnologies bring ingredients to the skin that work in ways unheard of five years ago.

Women often say to me, "My mother used only cold cream on her face, and her skin was fabulous." Truth to tell, *my* mother used only cold cream, and her mother before her. Genetics has a lot to do with good skin, and so does daily moisturizing, whatever you use. But good skincare has gotten beyond this. Way beyond. (Even Pond's, the good-old cold cream maker, is now using AHAs, retinol, and antioxidant vitamins in their Age Defying Complex.) We take advantage of technology in almost every aspect of our lives; why not go the high-tech route in beauty, as well?

Then there's the feeling that all products contain basically the same ingredients, so what's the sense in paying a lot. I'm not advocating that you spend a fortune, but major companies spend millions and devote decades of research into finding ingredients and systems they can patent. Meaning, you can't find exactly the same thing in a cheaper brand. And, obviously, you can't find some of the most costly ingredients in less-expensive brands, or they wouldn't be that price. You can be savvy, and **look for** key ingredients that exfoliate, hydrate, smooth, and brighten skin. And, whatever price you pay, check the package text for proprietary complexes and clinical trial research that substantiates the claims. Remember, a promise is a promise, but a percentage of improvement has to be proven!

## reality check: how much is a good thing?

Do you need thirty or forty ingredients in a product to do the job? Some companies will tell you that more is better. But, logic will tell you, more is more expensive. Estée Lauder herself was the first to explain that to women back in 1958, when she introduced Re-Nutriv Crème, the very first skincare product to cost $115 ($260 in today's money). It contained twenty-six ingredients, she explained in an ad headlined "What Makes a Cream Worth $115?" She also told women they were paying for the creativity of a company that could source and formulate twenty-six skin-improving ingredients and put them in a little jar.

That's still true. In 2002, the Estée Lauder Company developed Re-Nutriv's successor, with fifty-four ingredients. It's not just the crushed pearls from China for optical brightness that ups the costs. Re-Nutriv Ultimate Lifting Cream employs new biotechnologies to break up melanin deposits, combat ozone penetration, and strengthen cellular repair. Priced around $210, it's in the premiere tier of skincare products, but there are more expensive ones; there are also less-expensive products. It's the ingredients, and the technology behind them, that make the difference.

Clarins boasts forty-two natural ingredients in its Total Double Sérum, a dual-

• **Clarins Line Prevention Multi-Active Night Cream** works on irritation and inflammation, as well as skin's nighttime thirst.

• **Dior Phenomen-A Nuit** brings double retinol treatment to brighten and even the complexion, working on wrinkles while you sleep.

• **Lancôme Absolue Night** is a recovery treatment for face, throat, and décolleté, putting the power of wild yam, soy, and sea algae to work to help replenish skin and restore elasticity.

• **L'Oréal Plenitude Age Perfect Night** combines skin-whitening agents scutellaria and mulberry extracts with a patented beta hydroxy acid complex to renew skin overnight. Tightens and hydrates skin with vitamins E, B5 and B3.

• **Clinique Repairwear Intensive Night Cream** helps defuse skin stress and mend the look of lines and wrinkles.

and seal in extra moisture, plumping up skin cells. Nothing reconstructive happens; you wash them off, you wash away the plump. But don't ignore them; they'll provide a nice little lift while they're on. **look for** ingredients ranging from ceramides to soy proteins, antioxidants to hydrating lipids; they're very good to the skin.

*Town & Country*'s Janet Carlson Freed believes being too gaunt makes you look older. "Your fat has fallen away from your cheeks, so put some weight back on." She also has welcome, no-nonsense advice for improving glow, too:

## "Get some sleep."

Sleeplessness can be responsible for pallor. Women in perimenopause or menopause often have interrupted sleep, she points out, and "it shows up on your skin."

Shakespeare had it only partly right when he said that sleep "knits up the ravelled sleave of care." It also knits up the ravages of daytime environmental stress on your face. The skin restores and repairs itself at night (when it doesn't have any defending to do). It's quite busy as you sleep, correcting what it can. Which is why night creams are now more than moisturizing "goo." Many contain energy-supplying ingredients to help skin do its nocturnal job of recovery and renewal. Estée Lauder's Advanced Night Repair was one of the first products on the market—and is still one of the top-selling ones—to address the natural repair cycle of the skin; but now any skin-care line worth its salt has a night cream, each promising to tackle restoration while you sleep in its own way. Check out the Shopbox.

**the unwrinkle wonders** Yes, you can fill in a wrinkle by plumping, too, but there are better ways. Long before Retin-A was a flicker in the beauty industry's collective eye, dermatologists were using it to treat acne. And it worked. Along the way, it seemed to smooth out the skin, as well. Now retinol, a nonprescriptive derivative of vitamin A, has proven to be quite effective at minimizing wrinkling. In the bargain, it also evens skin tone, stimulates the production of collagen, restores skin clarity, lessens discoloration, re-

> **If your skin shows signs of flattening out, here's some advice you probably never expected to hear from a beauty editor: Gain a little weight.**

duces pore size, and amplifies moisture content. All over time, of course. Sound too good to be true? "The reason that retinol has persisted all this time is that it works," dermatologist Lydia Evans says.

Although retinol can sometimes irritate, skincare companies have been quick to develop lower concentrations, as well as time-release formulas, to deliver it gradually, and more gently, to the skin. The original Retin-A, and certain later-generation retinoids, are available only through a dermatologist, but gentler retinol can now be found in a multitude of cosmetics, moisturizers, cleansers, eye creams, and night creams. The concentration (and potency-protective packaging) is all-important to assure effectiveness, but unfortunately the percentage of active retinol is rarely noted on an over-the-counter product. And the manufacturers won't tell you, even if you call up and ask! In general, between 0.04 and 0.07 percent can produce results over several weeks, but even lower percentages can deliver benefits if used consistently.

L'Oréal suggests round-the-clock retinol action, with Line Eraser—an SPF 15 formula for daytime use, a concentrate for nightly renewal, and an A.M. and P.M. application of Line Eraser Eye to reduce the appearance of crinkles, wrinkles, and crow's feet. It's a twenty-four-hour assault, delivered in gentle, skin-friendly doses.

Still, there are women who would rather not use retinol. Admittedly, it can cause some tingling and redness when you first start to use it. "If you don't feel it, it probably isn't working," says Dr. Evans. "A few seconds of tingling is okay, but there's a big difference between slight tingling and burning." If your skin simply doesn't tolerate retinol, do not despair; there are other ways to address wrinkle formation. They go back to shoring up the skin's support system, but new technologies delve even deeper.

Back to the cells, again. Or, more specifically, cellular communication. Cells "talk" to one another all the time, through sophisticated, complex, and well-orchestrated processes. A large family of glycoproteins, called integrins, is primarily responsible for mediating direct cell-to-cell recognition and interaction, synchronizing the skin's signaling mechanisms. When the lines of communication are open, collagen, elastin, and laminin—elongated protein structures that help skin keep its shape—are produced in sufficient amounts. When some integrins disconnect, however, the skin's support network is compromised. Estée Lauder's Perfectionist Correcting Serum contains a patent-pending technology that works to reactivate integrins to help keep skin fully operational. Complete with light diffusion opticals and polymers, the serum blurs and fills fine lines from day one, improving skin radiance in the process. By addressing both internals and externals, Lauder's Perfectionist aims to lessen the lines you've got and prevent deeper furrows from forming.

The newest front on the war against wrinkles is relaxation. That's right. Just tell your wrinkles to relax! BOTOX started it all by inducing immobility of the skin muscles that, repetitively contracted, cause expression lines. Now Lancôme has developed a do-it-yourself relaxer. Their Résolution D-Contraxol Intensive Anti-Wrinkle Treatment works on the same anticontraction principle as BOTOX. The difference is, it operates at the cellular, not muscular, level to relax the tightened contractile fibers within the fibroblasts (cells that contribute to the formation of connective tissue fibers), and, in turn, the skin itself. This lessens the deep wrinkles, as the product smoothes and fills in fine lines with a web of polyamide fibers.

L'Oréal utilizes *Boswellia serrata* extract and manganese in a phyto-complex they call Boswelox™ to reduce the appearance of lines caused by microcontractions of the skin. Their Wrinkle De-Crease Advanced Wrinkle Corrector is a moisturizing cream formulated to soften frown lines, crow's feet, and deepening expression lines as it helps fight dehydration. There's optical help, as well. Polyamide fibers fill in lines, and laponite (tiny positively and negatively charged particles) forms a microscopic network on top of the skin to diffuse imperfections even more. L'Oréal recommends a special massaging application, to relax facial muscles and optimize effectiveness.

Now that skin-care science has gone beyond the surface of the skin, it's all become very complex. Fibroblasts. Cell signaling. Contractile fibers. But, basically, it's all about bump, dump, and plump, with products that are advanced enough to get the job done. While you don't have to stock your shelves with the most expensive ones on the market, you should at least keep up. **Look for** ingredients that are targeted to specific problems, and try new products that can work at a deeper level to optimize and energize the skin. You're going to see results. It may take some time; nothing happens overnight. But you will be giving your skin what it needs to function at a better level.

### glow with the flow For

those of us who can't wait for biology to take over, there are products that provide an instant glow. Fortunately, we are living in the new Age of Enlightenment. Luminosity is the latest wrinkle, pardon the expression, in the beauty game. Once reserved for pigmented makeup, new ways of adding light and color to the face now are avail-

## shopbox

• **L'Oreal Age Perfect Skin Illuminator & Age Spot Diffuser** contains light-reflecting ingredients that help brighten skin, while minimizing the appearance of brown spots and other discolorations. Formulated with beta hydroxy acid to accelerate cell turnover, and ingredients to encourage even-toned, luminous-looking skin.

• **Dior Eclat Parfait Total Radiance,** a rosy gel to use after treatment and before foundation to smooth and brighten skin, relieving "signs of tiredness."

• **Biotherm Pure Bright Illuminating Essence** rids skin of dulling impurities with a blend of lactic and glycolic acids, then polishes it to perfection with light-reflecting minerals.

• **Georgette Klinger Instant Radiance Facial Renewing Balm,** a creamy pick-me-up lotion for those times when your complexion needs a boost: before a night out, after a late night, times

(continued on next page)

when your skin looks "tired," just about any time. Formulated with anti-irritants, vitamins, and moisturizers, it combats skin fatigue to refresh and brighten. Can be worn alone or under your normal moisturizer.

• **Dior Capture R-Flash Instant Ultra-Smoothing Fluid,** a complexion evener that smoothes wrinkles and fine lines, restoring brightness in the process.

able in treatment products as well as color cosmetics. They offer a way to feel good about your skin without having to wear much makeup at all.

The trick is called optical technology. It's a way of changing what the eye sees, either through scattering light, or changing the color of the light. When you scatter the light, you blur the image (and the wrinkles), rather than highlighting it. Reflectivity has been with the beauty world since the invention of "frosted" colors. But today's illumination goes far beyond glittery flecks; it changes the actual color of the light. Microscopic crystals break down white light into different color components, absorbing certain spectrums of UV light to correct skin tone, or emitting color of their own.

Buying treatment products today is like a quick trip to the jewelry counter. Estée Lauder's Light Source utilizes the tiniest particles of Brazilian emerald to neutralize excessive redness, especially good for younger skin, twenty-seven to forty. Resilience Lift, Estée Lauder's day and night moisturizers for skin that shows signs of "hormonal aging," contains chroma-brighteners to impart a rosy glow. Other gem-of-an-idea lotions contain tourmaline (Aveda), diamond powder (La Mer), crushed pearls (Re-Nutriv Ultimate Lifting Cream), and optical pearls (L'Oréal Age Perfect).

In addition to light-reflecting particles, silicone polymers change the optics of an area, as well as fill in the lines to provide a velvety, seamless texture. This is what some companies call "refinishing" the skin. The texture is indeed transformed; skin becomes unbelievably smooth and soft at first application. Estée Lauder's Idealist and Perfectionist products offer two good examples of instant refinishing with polymers.

No matter how they add the light, a multitude of skin-care products are out there, ready and waiting to hit the high beams on your skin. See the Shopbox for others.

Optical technology is instant gratification. If you use treatment products that boost luminosity, your skin will snap out of its doldrums. If you use makeup with light-reflecting micropowders, you'll have the lightness and glow that gives your face an instant lift. If you use both, layering an optical moisturizer *and* a light-reflecting makeup, "better have a friend check you out before you walk out the door," warns Janet Carlson Freed. "A little sleight of hand is fine. Too much, and you'll look like Sparkle Plenty."

# NINE

# great face: getting makeup right

**Keep cosmetics sheer and light, with a dash of reflectivity.**

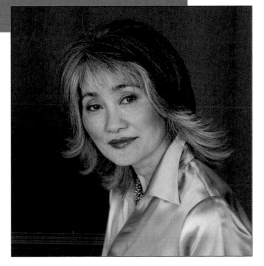

When you take care of your skin first, it's going to change the way you think about makeup. You're not going to be looking for heavy cover, bolder colors, and things you've never worn before. Face it, too much makeup can look garish near a paler shade of hair. The contrast is completely unnatural. Too little, and you run the risk of fading away. There's a happy medium in there somewhere, and it may have to do with simply changing the palette of colors you normally use. Or learning new techniques of applying color. It's certainly fun to experiment—with a light hand. But even if you're not a "makeup person," there are lots of ways to add a natural bit of color and glow to your skin.

**the glow-getters** Now that you've seen how skincare products come with varying degrees of illumination, you might expect cosmetics to

## shopbox

• **Estée Lauder Go Tan.** A self-tanning collection for a year-round glow. In new, no-drip Towelettes for Body and Face, a Sunless Spray that spritzes on from any angle, a Fast Tan Quick Dry Sunless Spray, and Body Shimmer (a sunscreen with a touch of sparkle).

• **Clinique Body Quick Bronze Self-Tanner.** Tinted, so you can lay down color and see where it goes before the self-tanning starts.

• **Clinique Self Tanning Body Mist** A lightweight, oil-free, alcohol-free spray that lets you spritz on sun, developing a tan in two to three hours.

• **L'Oréal Ombrelle Sunless Spray SPF 12,** with a 360-degree pump, sprays on easily for complete coverage. Provides sunscreen protection in medium and dark shades.

• **Estée Lauder Sunless Stay Bronze Moisturizing Tan** develops a golden glow with low-level tanners, then keeps skin smooth.

supply the same. They do. New forms of sheer, translucent makeup also provide a glow. Light-refracting formulations impart color and light to minimize lines, and won't dull down your complexion.

"Anything that is heavy, matte, or powdery is going to be an age adder," says Lois Joy Johnson, beauty and fashion director of *More* magazine. If what you're using now seems that way, she advises blending a drop of moisturizer with your base to sheer the color, and skip the powder altogether. If your moisturizer happens to contain a bit of reflectivity, you've just turned your foundation optical!

A generation or two ago, it seemed the older a woman got, the more powder she used. A "shiny nose" was to be avoided at all costs. Today, however, glowing skin is equated with youth and vitality, and powders often come in creamy formulations, or have an element of reflectivity. And that's all for the good, according to makeup expert and principal makeup artist for this book Jennifer Wobito. "Don't be afraid to shine," she says. "Shine is extremely lively, and it brings everything out—your eyes, your lips. It's like your hormones are working."

## go for the bronze

Bronzers—self-tanners or makeup products—win rave reviews from women with gray hair, especially now that you can find shades that don't contrast too strongly with fair-colored skin, or a whiter shade of hair. These products can deliver natural, week-at-the-beach color without a "made-up" look. One word of warning: don't go off half-baked. If your face has a sun-kissed glow, any other visible skin should, too. Don't forget the back of your hands, legs, décolletage. And, whatever you do, don't forget to exfoliate your skin before you self-tan. You've got to smooth the surface for the smoothest, most even results.

## all-over self-tanners

They've come a long way from the "agent oranges" of yore. Today's formulations are easier to apply, kind to the skin, and deliver a truer tan color. The easiest ones to apply provide a tint all their own, for instant gratification. The tint also guides your hand to avoid streaking while you stroke it on. You know where it is, you know where it isn't. But today's formulations have been developed to be "streak free," and they go on the body in a variety of different ways: a mist, a spritz, a towelette. It's a little more carefree, not the painstaking process it was before. Look to the Shopbox for some of the best.

## just-the-face sunless

**tanners** Tanners especially formulated for the face put gentle color where you want it most, and where you want the sun least. UV radiation is the direct cause of photoaging, and it slows down the cells' own immune response. Translation: While you're out there wrecking your skin, your cells can't effectively repair it. If you want your face to tan, the safest way is letting it do it itself, with products that provide the additional benefits of daily skincare as

### shopbox

• **L'Oréal Ombrelle Sunless Tanning Cream for Face SPF 15** solves the problem of applying sunscreen while using a sunless tanner. One step to healthy-looking color and sun protection. In tinted and nontinted formulas. The bronzing tint gives a glow of color while developing, so you can see where you apply it for even coverage.

• **Clarins Radiance-Plus,** a moisture-rich cream-gel for face, neck, and décolleté, is formulated with tan boosters and a unique vitamin complex to keep skin soft and glowing. Brings a natural, outdoorsy radiance to the complexion almost instantly.

• **Clinique Face Quick Bronze Tinted Self-Tanner** for see-as-you-glow application. Provides an instant sun-warmed look, a tan in a few hours.

## shopbox

• **Jergens Soft Shimmer,** a body moisturizer infused with mica titanium dioxide, for an all-over body glow.

• **Prescriptives Sunsheen Body Tint** is a prismatic gel that refracts and reflects the light, imparting a soft, golden glow to the skin.

• **Jergens Ash Relief Moisturizer,** formulated with beta hydroxy, cocoa butter, and shea butter, to banish dry, flaky skin, and moisturize at the same time.

• **L'Oréal HydraFresh Express Super-Light Moisturizing Body Spray** swooshes on microscopic droplets of vitamin-packed oil in a rejuvenating spray application. Boosted with vitamins E and C to combat free radicals, and moisturizing vitamin $B_5$, it leaves skin conditioned and quenched for twenty-four hours.

well as protection against the sun. Look for some of the best facial self-tanners in the Shopbox.

## the body beautiful

When you've got a good glow going all over, there are lots of ways to keep it that way. Look to products that deliver good moisturization, along with a little glow of their own. Be sure to see the Shopbox.

## naked without foundation?

If you feel that way, there is probably a reason. As we age, our complexions become uneven, splotchy. Tiny broken capillaries, sun damage, and age spots can make for a road map surface. Amazingly, this is precisely the time many women choose not to wear foundation. Revlon, who did a study of such things in the late 1990s, found that more and more women were dropping out of the foundation category in their thirties, forties, and fifties. Why? Cheryl Vitali, executive vice president and general manager of Revlon, Global, at that time, offers two reasons: (1) Women were no longer getting the same results from their foundation that they got when their skin was younger. (2) Foundation is the hardest to buy, apply, and get right. Women were too busy to deal with this, so they gave up. "Skincare and treatment products were also on the rise," she says. "Sales in these categories were going up as foundation sales were plummeting. When women started taking better care of their skin, there was less of a need to cover it up."

This presented an interesting challenge to Vitali, and, along with her product development and marketing team, she set about to create a simplified nonfoundation product. The result? Revlon Skinlights. "What it did was to give women light and glow, without promising flawless skin. Everyone promised flawless skin. We wanted to give women easy-to-buy color, without coverage, without moisturizer, without all the bells and whistles. There were no antiaging claims. Only an instant illumination."

Color selection became simpler with Skinlights. There are only about half a dozen shades. None are meant to match the skin; the transparency makes it adaptable to practically any skin tone. "You can't really go far wrong," says Vitali, "and if you decide the shade you buy is too dark, you can save it for summer." Revlon's Skinlights collection includes a Face Illuminator lotion, a quick-to-slick-on stick, a powder, and an Illusion Wand concealer with its own little brush that nicely diffuses light away from wrinkles.

If your skin is very pale, and you don't like a lot of color, you can still add a bit of luminosity, at selected spots, or all over. **look for** sheer, glow-only highlighters that provide just a hint of glisten and tint (pearl, gold, a slight pink) without a lot of heavy-handed color. See what we mean in the Shopbox.

## shopbox

• **Revlon Skinlights Natural Light** highlighter, an almost clear, natural glow in stick form.

• **Smashbox Artificial Light,** a lotion light diffuser to use alone or mix with foundation in shades like Diffuse, Glare, Glow, and Reflect.

• **Lorac's Luminizer,** in Pearl or Gold, for a fast, sheer swipe of light.

• **Neutrogena Shimmer Sheers,** tubes of transparent gleam for cheeks, lips, and eyes. Formulated with aloe vera and vitamins.

• **Magic by Prescriptives Illuminating Liquid Potion** is a holographic liquid with three-dimensional pigments made of spherical, multilayered particles that change the way skin reflects light, perfecting surface appearance and providing a youthful glow.

**sun makeup = un-makeup** If you don't want to self-tan, but do want a warm glow, there are lots of ways to add a bit of sunny color without feeling like you're wearing serious makeup at all. There are intriguing new formulations that go beyond the deep, dark blushers that used to stand for bronzers. Now you can spray it on, brush it on, rub it on, dab it on cheeks, or add it to your mois-

**143**

• **Estée Lauder's Amber Bronze** collection, with Bronzing Powder, Cool Bronze Loose Powder, and Liquid Bronzer for Face. In a wide range of shades for even the fairest complexions, the products deliver a skin-smoothing benefit.

• **Lancôme Star Bronzer** collection offers Magic Golden Spray, an "instant" shimmer of sun; a Magic Bronzing Brush that swivels up luminous color at the press of a button; and a compact bronzing powder.

• **Lancôme's Sheer Glow Fluid Highlighter** gives a sheer, shimmerless sunkissed look.

• **Clinique City Block Sheer Shimmer Oil-Free Daily Face Protector SPF 15,** for a natural glow that feels makeup-free, with just a hint of shimmer. A sheer, light, natural glow with UVA/UVB and antioxidant protection. In two shades.

• **Clinique City Block Sheer Tint Oil-Free Daily Face Protector SPF 15** adds a hint of tint to the sheer summer look, along with UVA/UVB and antioxidant protection. Delicate
*(continued on next page)*

turizer. It just depends how you like your glow-to-go. The Shopbox will give you a good list of tan-in-the-can products.

**the base line** For coverage that evens skin tone, dispels flaws, and gives skin a finished look, you want foundation. Not the makeup mask of old, foundation today is lightweight, adjustable to skin type, and as natural-looking as you want. While it's trickier to get right than transparent tints, set some rules for yourself. The first rule is comfort. How does it feel on your skin? You have to wear it all day. If you're satisfied with the texture, **look for** three things only: (1) Its level of coverage (sheer to full). (2) The amount of nurturing skincare it supplies. (3) The finish you like (matte to luminous). Put it all together, and what have you got? According to Lois Joy Johnson, a sheer, moisturizing, light-reflecting foundation helps skin look as dewy and fresh as possible.

Now it's time to select the shade. You know the first rule: Stay close to your skin tone. Foundation should never be used to boost your color, or turn you any shade you aren't. If a certain shade worked for you pre-gray, it's probably still your best bet, or one very close to it. Noted makeup artist Ramy Gafni says, "Your foundation shouldn't have to change just because you are gray."

One thing to be wary of, however, is anything too pink; it can lead to the Mrs. Santa

Claus syndrome. If your skin has a natural flush, or a red undertone, it's going to make you look redder, not healthier, not rosier, not younger. If your skin is sallow, it's never going to look natural. It's best to stick with neutral tones ("they give you more leeway," says Gafni). And don't think you automatically have to go to "cooler" shades, he advises.

"Most women perceive their skin tone as being paler than it is," says *More*'s Lois Joy Johnson, "and they select a foundation shade that is too pink, chalky, or artificial-looking." Women are also often unmindful of their décolleté. "Most women over forty have some degree of sun damage on their chest," says Johnson. "The skin there is usually a deeper color than the face. You want to be able to create a natural, seamless effect." When women with darker complexions select a shade that is too light, the effect is just as unsettling. The face looks masklike, and can appear ashy, especially if the skin is dry.

## accent colors: the danger zone

Getting your skin color right is only the beginning. After that, it gets trickier. It's far easier to go wrong with the accent colors you choose for blush, eyeshadow, and lipstick, and yet these are the shades that most define your face. The whole color cosmetic world of pinks and reds and corals and lavenders and teals and blues spins in front of your eyes. The gleaming, glossy, velvety, or matte

color in light-to-medium and medium-to-dark formulations.

- **Clinique's Colour Rub Allover Lustre** has the right touch of transparency for a natural sunlight effect. To use as a blush or a highlighter in four shades: Nude Luster, Rose Luster, Sheer Radiance, and Bronze Glow.

- **Clarins Bronzing Powder Duo** provides two sheer, luminous bronzing powder shades in a single compact for a natural, healthy glow.

- **Bobbi Brown's Bronzer/Blush Compact Duo** doubles up as well with a cheeky bronze and pink combination.

- **Dior's Terra Bella,** a velvety-textured powder, leaves a matte light-reflecting finish to brighten an existing tan, or add a healthy summer look to skin.

- **MD Skincare All-in-One Tinted Moisturizer SPF 15** adds subtle, sheer color to all-day hydration and UV protection. More a daily foundation alternative than a bronzer, it gives skin a soft touch of color that nicely supports a richer bronzing blush. Choose from light, medium, and dark.

145

shades beckon from every cosmetics counter. They seduce in the prettiest rainbow of ways. There's danger here. One way to go wrong is to intensify everything, using more color than you ever have in your life. Another way is to make poor color choices.

> "Gray hair itself is a strong feature. You don't want your makeup to compete with your hair. A little mascara and a bright lipstick might be enough."
> *Ramy Gafni, Makeup Artist*

"I used to feel like I wanted to use color all the time," says Skinklinic's Kathy Dwyer, "but now I don't. By day I don't use anything on my face because my skin tone is even and fresh. By night, I might use it, and have fun with it. Wearing the latest 'style' in makeup is a nighttime event. During the day, you just want to look good and pulled together."

Her advice is simply to accent areas of the face that you want to enhance. "Find your best feature, and then make sure it's your best feature by taking care of it. Then, and only then, enhance it with color cosmetics."

**changing your colors** Two things can happen with graying hair: (1) You may have to totally rethink your palette of makeup accent colors. (2) You many need only to adjust them slightly. Let's start with Case 1: Why does your lifelong palette no longer work? If you've always liked yellow-based tones, for instance—the golden amber blushes, the orangey lipsticks—they may look deadly in the presence of silver or white hair. Remember, the perception of your skin tone may change without a surrounding frame of color. You may have been able to wear certain shades before because your hair reflected the right tonality all around your face. Minus that, you may realize your skin is not tawny, but pinky-fair; not amber but sallow. A silvery shade to your hair reflects a cooler tonality as well, and this can compound the "changing skin tone" appearance.

This happened to Mary Louise Farrell, a woman who continued to wear the right makeup for someone with fair skin and auburn hair long after the color had faded. "I had changed my wardrobe, but I was still wearing the same makeup. I used to wear all the coral-based shades, and I later found out they were so wrong for me. With white hair, it became more obvious that my coloring was blue-based, so I switched to cooler colors, and the first time I wore them and went to work, everyone said, 'Wow!' "

Case 2: Adjustments can be made. Say you have yellow undertones to your skin and silvery hair. It's like mixing metals. Part silver, part gold. Do you play to your hair, or your skin tone? Yes. You have to do a little of both. Don't abandon completely foundation and accent colors that have golden tones in them. Just cool them down a bit. A soft, warm beige instead of a sun-kissed honey or tawny foundation shade, for instance. Switch from an amber blush to an earthy rose, or a dusty peach. Take your lip color from copper/coral to cranberry, or a good beige rose. Just cool it. But don't, *don't* think you're suddenly Snow White. If you change your palette completely, and go for magenta lips, clear pink blush, and a little blue on the eyes, you'll clash with your own skin tone.

**forever red** There's nothing more striking with salt-and-pepper hair or an icy shade of white. A clear red delivers the most impact, but a very slightly spiced red or a blue-red may go better with your skin tone. Think in terms of an apple, burgundy, or berry red. Darker complexions can go to the deep, rich plums, but don't go too dark. A slash of dark lipstick is instantly aging (especially if your lips are thinning—they'll look even thinner). If you

> **"If your cheek color is warm, keep your lips warm. If your cheek color is cool, then the lips should be cool, too."**
> **Jennifer Wobito, principal makeup artist for Going Gray, Looking Great!**

like a deeper shade, brighten it by buying it in a glossier, liquid form that sends back light, or pick the shade you like in a lip pencil, fill the color in lightly, then dot a bit of clear or lightly tinted gloss over. A *bit*. Gooey is for kids. You want a fresh, moist, natural-looking mouth that adds a little brightness to your face. Nothing more, nothing less.

**expert advice:** Who says you have to play it cool, all the way? Or use only warm shades? Makeup pro Ramy Gafni says mixing adds a nice surprise. And your eye color will give you a clue to shade selection. For instance, blue eyes generally signal a cooler palette. But you can warm up the eyes with golden taupe shades. With dark brown eyes, the reverse works. Darker skin tones can do cool, smoky eyes, and richer colors everyplace else; a good burgundy on the lips. The going rule: bolder eyes/softer lips. And vice versa.

### know when to say "help!" When your hair color

changes (one way or the other!), it's time to try new makeup shades. But where to start? There are so many colors out there today, so many tints of color, so many textures and so many formulas that searching for the right ones can be intimidating to some women. Or overwhelming—the needle-in-the-haystack feeling.

*Do* go to a line representative, or a brand-affiliated makeup artist. *Don't* feel you have to buy everything they suggest, or even anything at all. Women always feel they "have to" buy something when a makeup artist spends time with them. It's not required. Go to the counter of a brand you like and may already use; you'll be more comfortable with the products. And you won't mind picking up one or two things while you're there, if you feel you simply must. Time and time again, women told me it was an "expert" who figured it out for them, and they were so pleased, they continued to wear the shades "forever."

John Barrett, owner of the John Barrett Salon at Bergdorf Goodman, suggests you see a makeup expert once a year to review what's right for you.

> "You know how good you feel when you clean out your closet and throw away any clothes that are no longer applicable to your life. The same thing is true with your makeup."

# the shade selector: the beauty experts come to you

To get you started, on the following pages you'll find eight perfect palettes of color, suggested by leading cosmetic companies just for *Going Gray, Looking Great!* Created specifically for various gray tonalities, eye color, and skin tone, these palette templates will help you customize your own color selections the next time you visit their counters.

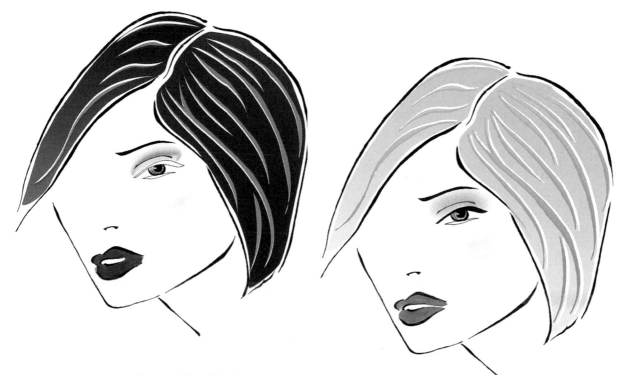

**Brunette Mélange/Olive Skin Tone/ Brown Eyes**
*Clinique* Touch Base for Eyes in Canvas, Pair of Shades Eye Shadow Duo in Ash Violets; Long Pretty Lashes Mascara in Black; Soft Pressed Powder Blusher in New Clover; Quickliner for Lips in Velvet Rose; Colour Surge Lipstick in Wild Berry

**Blonde Mélange/Fair Skin Tone/ Blue Eyes**
*Estée Lauder* Pure Color Eyeshadow in Tea Box; Liner: Artist's Eye Pencil in Brown Writer; Magnascopic Volumizing Mascara in Black; Amber Bronze Bronzing Powder (Medium Palette-Light Side); Pure Color Lipstick in Paradise Pink, or Pure Color Lip Vinyl in Plastique Pink

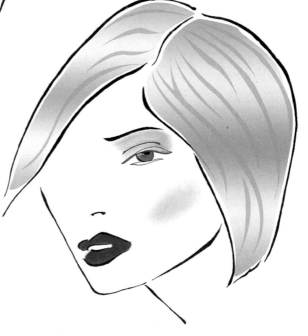

**Smoky Charcoal/Black Skin Tone/Brown Eyes**
*MAC* Eye Kohl in Smolder (lid); Eye Shadow in Folie (lid), Soft Brown (crease), Motif (brow bone), Carbon (lash line); Pro Lash Mascara in Coal Black; Raisinesque Cheekhue; Pencil in Mahogany (lip liner); Lipstick in Rage

**Sterling/Fair Skin Tone/Blue Eyes**
*L'Oréal* Wear Infinité Eye Shadow Duo in Berry Pinks; Le Grand Kohl Eye Liner in Smoke; Lash Out Mascara in Black; Feel Naturale Powder Blush in Mauvelous; Endless Lipcolour in Perfect Plum

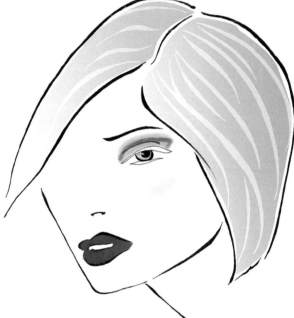

**Silver/Fair Skin Tone/Blue Eyes**
*Clinique* Touch Base for Eyes in Canvas; Pair of Shades Eye Shadow Duo in Pink Chocolates; Lash Doubling Mascara in Brown; Soft Pressed Powder Blusher in Pink Blush; Quickliner for Lips in Tawny Tulip; Colour Surge Lipstick in Toasted Rose

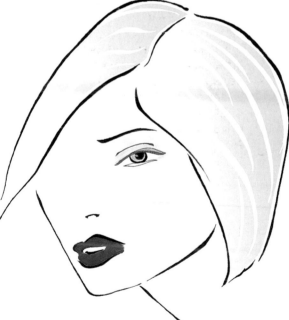

**Pearl/Honey Skin Tone/Brown Eyes**
*Clarins* Eye Colour Trio in Zephyr 07; Eyeliner Pencil in Grey 02; Pure Volume Mascara in Pure Black 02; Multi-Blush in Tender Lichee 01 (cream blush) or Powder Blush in Heather Pink 20; Lip Liner in Natural Brown 02; Le Rouge Lipstick in Illusion 230

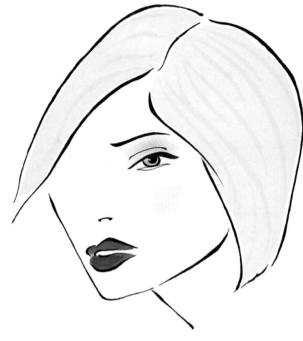

**Snow/Tawny Skin Tone/Green Eyes**
*Estée Lauder* Pure Color Eyeshadow in
Mocha Cup; Liner: Artist's Eye Pencil in
Slate Writer; Illusionist Maximum Curling
Mascara in Black; Amber Bronze Bronzing
Powder (Medium Palette-Light Side); Pure
Color Lipstick in Bronze Idol, or Pure Color
Lip Vinyl in Wet Mango

**Ice/Amber Skin Tone/Hazel Eyes**
*Prescriptives* Quick Pick Eyeshadows in
Champagne, Buttercup, Apricot, Latte, Stormy;
Deluxe Eye Pencil in Charcoal, Midnight; False
Eyelashes Plush Mascara in Plush Black; Powder
Cheekcolor in Cinnamon, Pompeii; Deluxe Lip
Pencil in Hazel; Incredible Lipcolor in Champagne;
Lippity Split in Taffy

**raising eyebrows** The single most important accent area for women with gray, white, or silver-touched hair, by unanimous decision, is the eyebrows. Contrast seems to be key; they won't leave home without it. The eyebrows tend to gray later than the rest of your hair, so Mother Nature does a good job of providing contrast. But sometimes the effect is more startling than simpatico. Black, black brows against white, white hair and pale, pale skin can get a little Groucho Marx. Your brows have always gone with your hair before, and they should now. But women continue to pluck stray grays with a fervor. Should you?

When I worked with makeup artist Rex Hilverdink on the book *Forever Beautiful,* specifically for women over forty, he was adamant that lighter brows are more youthful; it's the contrast itself that is aging. If your hair frames your face with a lighter color, there's a softening effect, and anything too dark on your face can simply look harsh.

Kathy Dwyer agrees. "There can't be too much contrast. If they're dark, with graying starting to show, you could use a blonde pencil or a taupe pencil over them. You can make them pronounced, with a good line to them without making them the most contrasting thing on your face. Use eyebrow pencil; it's easiest. Or investigate permanent makeup, which implants soft micropigments into the upper layers of the skin, for the lash line or brows. But find a really good person to do it. This isn't the kind of thing you go to a tattoo parlor for!"

"No black," says Ramy Gafni. "When you choose an eyebrow pencil, look for a neutral shade that is only one shade darker than the color of your gray hair. Taupe generally works best."

Jennifer Wobito also advises against black and likes concrete and slate shades, preferably powder eye shadows, not pencils, for more natural blending. "They're still ashy," she says, "and the tonality complements gray hair." But you have to be careful here. "Some women say, 'I have gray hair, so let me use a gray pencil.' In certain lights, this can look blue."

John Barrett believes eyebrows are "crucial" for all women, especially when they're going through changes in the color of their hair. "Your eyebrows have to change; you should have an eyebrow adjustment on an annual basis, correcting the shape and the color. It's all about grooming," he says.

## shopbox

• **Clarins Instant Light Perfecting Touch,** a brush-on concealer that uses illumination to perfect any emergency like dark circles, fine lines, and signs of skin fatigue.

• **Clinique Airbrush Concealer** provides illumination with correction and makes application all the easier with its self-filling brush wand.

Of course, it's best to deplump eyes with proper treatment, morning and night. Three to try:

• **Clarins Extra-Firming Eye Contour Serum** does a 24/7 attack on aging, or can be used at any time to smooth and brighten surface skin, and give crow's-feet the boot. It actually dries like a powder, preventing color slip-off.

• **L'Oréal Visible Results Eye** combines tightening technologies with light diffusion. Formulated to smooth first lines and brighten skin with optical diffusers, vitamin C, and caffeine.

• **L'Oréal Age Perfect Eye** with vitamin E, shea butter, and apricot oil, provides intense moisture, as brightening botanicals such as ruscusaculatus, a root extract, work with light diffusers to help diminish the appearance of dark circles.

When eyebrows start to gray, he advises having them professionally colored, then using makeup to shade grow-ins between appointments. There are also very good mascara-like wands especially for eyebrows that can add a touch of color, or simply enhance the brow's natural sheen. **look for** Chanel Brow Shaper, Maybelline Brow Styling Gel in Clear, Taupe, and Brunette, and Dior's Gel Fixateur Brow Gel. These are great to define, shape, and hold brows (and color!) in place, using short upward strokes from the eye end of the brow outward. If you're using a colored product, take a tip from the way colorists blend in a minimum amount of gray hair, and select a shade lighter than your natural brow color to soften the effect.

Pale blonde brows need more definition, and a little more artistry. A two-pencil trick will work better for you. Lightly feather alternating strokes of light taupe and blonde, then top with a clear brow gel to set and hold the line.

## lighten up the excess baggage

Nothing takes attention away from a perfect brow more than a deep dark circle under the eyes. Okay, a bag. A little illumination comes to the rescue here. Newer than thick camouflage creams or "cover-up" sticks, today's concealers and eye treatment products blend lightness (in formulation) and light (in optics) to soften the appearance of bags, sags, and shadows. See the Shopbox on the previous page for the kind of camouflage that will get you out of the dark ages.

## don't step on the cracks

If you've got 'em, you know where they are. Around the eyes. On the lids. Prancing around the lip line. Tiny little creases can play havoc with any color product you apply. Your shade will settle in these lines, or "feather" into them. That's why lipsticks bleed, eye shadow disappears, and color collects. It's worse if you use a high-sparkle shade. You're just adding tinsel to wrinkles.

### Eye Shadow

If your eyelids are what they call "crepey," less is more. You can use a color shadow, if you like, but keep it light in application and tone. "If the skin around your eyes isn't smooth, this can be very dangerous," says John Barrett. "You don't want to be loading something on there. You don't want anything that just sits on the skin."

Far better simply to highlight the firmer brow bone area just under your brows, and let your skin's natural shadows define the crease. If you want to add color, lid preps are great for this. They provide a smoother surface to the lid, and blot up any oils that cause color to move. "Powder eye

## shopbox

• **Georgette Klinger Take Cover Eyelid Foundation,** a silky brightener, evens skin tone like a good foundation should, and minimizes the appearance of fine lines with optical diffusers and tighteners. You can smooth just a bit on up to the brow, and it will dry into a smooth finish. Use it with eye shadow, and the color will go on smoother, without creasing or fading. Or use it alone for a soft, natural, smooth finish.

• **Clinique Touch Base for Eyes** in a neutral Canvas shade, holds eye shadow without creasing, and helps it last longer.

• **Revlon Illuminance Eye Cream** is not technically a primer, but it adds sheer soft luster to the lids to diffuse light, and put creases into soft focus.

• **Dior Light and Lasting Eyeshadow in Beige Veil,** not a primer, either, but a good creamy neutral with slight shimmer that helps to brighten the area, without putting it on auto flash.

shadows blow right off skin when the surface isn't smooth, so you never get true color," says Eileen Paley, senior vice president of product development and marketing for Georgette Klinger. "That's why it's better to have a perfectly primed lid." For new products that pave the way to a smoother, color-holding lid surface, see the Shopbox.

> **Beauty Editor Tip: "You can add shape to the eyes without a hard line. Use muted neutral tones like grays, camels, browns, close to the lash line."**
> *Lois Joy Johnson, beauty and fashion director, More magazine*

### Eyeliner

Like the definition of a little line at the base of the lashes? Maybe it's time to rethink that. If you have darkness or discoloration under your eyes, a line at your lower lashes only draws attention to it. Say good-bye to the black liquid liner, too. It's harsh (read: aging) and takes a very steady hand. Even if you apply with perfect stability, a liquid can leave an uneven line if the surface of the skin is wrinkled. It's kind of like falling between the cracks. The result: a series of dots and dashes instead of a smooth, subtle line. Instead, opt for a pencil or powder eye shadow (often much easier to apply to fragile skin) that you can stroke on with a cotton swab, or slant-edged small brush. You can smudge it for a softer look—what magazines call a "smoky eye"—but be careful. Too smudged, and it just looks dirty.

If you're going to use pencils to line the eyes, make sure they're creamy, and don't pull or tug at the skin. Two I like are MAC Eye Kohl and Borghese Eye Accento Pencil, with its built-in sponge-tip smudger.

> **Beauty Editor Tip: "Take a moonlight shade and dab it just beside the bridge of your nose, where it tends to be dark. It's a great five P.M. pick-me-up, if you're going out after work."**
> *Janet Carlson Freed, beauty and health director, Town & Country*

### Blush

Any blush that simply lays on top of the skin is eventually going to sink into wrinkles. That's why cream formulations are better than powder. They blend easily, don't sink in, and deliver the bonus of a moist little glow as well. But work with what you find easiest to apply, because the net effect is all in the application. Whether you choose a cream, a stick, or a powder blush, go easy. Wearing too much blush to bring "life" to your face is as close to disaster as you can get with gray hair.

Blush placement becomes critical, too. Keep it farther away from the outside of your face than you used to. Don't blend it all the way to the hairline; feather it out well before it gets to the edge. You can bring it up a notch, especially if you're bothered by dark circles under your eyes. A bit of brighter color steals attention away from deep shadows. Instead of focusing on the "apple" of your cheeks, bring your glow *slightly* higher for a natural, sun-kissed effect. WARNING: Don't go near under-eye wrinkles or into the hollow, or you'll look like you need eight more hours of sleep.

> **Makeup Artist Tip: "I love the way golds look on eyes. Especially if the skin is thin on the lids, causing a purplish cast. Warm, golden tones around the eyes get rid of the shadowy look and brighten up the whole area."** *Jennifer Wobito, principal makeup artist,* Going Gray, Looking Great!

### Blending

Whatever colors you use on your face, and wherever you use them, the most important beauty technique is blending. The soft smudging of color, done by fingers, sponge, or brush, is the best way to integrate accent colors into a total, natural look. There should never be a sharp line of demarcation between cheeks and foundation, never a "layered look" on the eyelid. One shade should flow seamlessly into the next. You can go slightly darker and more dramatic at night, *if you blend*. You can stay with colors that are pretty close to your natural skin tone by day, *if you blend*. "It's all about making makeup a part of your skin," says Wobito.

### Lip Color

If your lips are "stitched" all around, it's best to smooth the surface first so lipstick is less likely to feather into crevices. Look for two of the best in the Shopbox. When you're ready to apply color, **look for** lipsticks that provide maximum

• **Clarins Extra-Firming Lip & Contour Care,** a lightweight, gel-like cream, adds a little "lift" to lip contours, as it visibly reduces fine lines on and around lips. Fortified with moisturizers like mango and hibiscus extracts, special soothers, antipollution vitamins and optical-correcting pigments, this nonoily formula helps lips appear smoother, fuller, and better defined. You can use it morning, evening, or as often as desired to aid lipstick application.

• **Georgette Klinger Anti-Aging Lip Treatment** Infused with rich moisturizers like shea butter, sunflower oil, and barrier-repairing ceramides to hydrate and hold moisture, plus antioxidant vitamins to protect against future damage, it helps "plump" lines on and around your lips. With fewer lines to sneak into, lipstick stays where it should.

color intensity in a moisture-rich formula. Preferably, all in one. High-pigment content can dry lips, so the more moisture in the formula, the better. Lips should have a little life to them; a flat, matte color will call attention to wrinkles and dryness because there's nothing to divert the eye.

"Glossy lips are so much more lively than dry, matte lips," says Jennifer Wobito. A moist mouth is simply more youthful. Just avoid the sparkly stuff, and go for a soft glow.

But be careful. Emollients, or oils, in the formula can make color move. Too much wetness, and color will head straight for the crinkles around the mouth. That's why, when you're using a very moist lip gloss, you should place it in the center of your lip, well away from the lip line. The waxy pigment of a lip liner pencil tends to corral color a bit, and now some lipsticks are using emollients that don't "travel," minimizing color slip. The Shopbox will tell you the ones that stay put, plus offer the right kind of care to keep lips moist, soft, and luminous.

## what happens when you smile?

No matter how artfully you apply your lipstick, sooner or later your lips will part, and your teeth will show. Once your hair turns gray, silver, or white, age-related dulling and discoloring of the teeth is more noticeable; there isn't that warmth of color in your hair to draw the eye away. In fact, the pure contrast of bright white hair can put your teeth to shame, making them look more off-color than ever. Rule of thumb: The whiter the hair goes, the whiter the teeth should be.

It's simply the best antiaging "cosmetic" you can buy.

Fortunately, today, there's so much you can do to bring teeth back to their youthful, natural shade, or whiten them a notch or two. When you consider a method, you should look first for the key whitening ingredient—either hydrogen peroxide or carbamide peroxide. The hydrogen peroxide works faster, but it's less stable, and only keeps its potency in vacuum-sealed packaging. Carbamide, the most common bleaching agent, is more stable, and therefore used in many more products you can buy off the shelves, but it can create an acidic environment that may irritate gums or cause tooth sensitivity.

Second, consider the way the whitening agents get to the teeth. Some systems are simply better at targeting teeth and providing the kind of contact time and peroxide strength that make a difference. Then take into account your teeth sensitivity, your patience level, and your pocketbook. Know the results you want to achieve, and discuss the options with your dentist (even if you're going to use a drugstore whitening product).

Armed with the right information, you can make a wise choice from a dentist-administered ARC lamp treatment; at-home tray or mouth guard systems; whitening strips; brush-on gels; and whitening toothpastes. Don't expect the most dramatic re-

## shopbox

• **Clinique Colour Surge Lipstick** for a full load of color (15 percent pigment, as opposed to the average 9 to 10 percent), with a creamy texture. It adds soft waxes, similar to those found in glosses, to traditional hard waxes, so you don't have the dried-out look that some high-pigment lipsticks can give you.

• **Clinique Moisture Sheer Lipstick SPF 15** averts a hard-edged lipstick look, with sheer, transparent color. Provides comfortable moisture as well as protection.

• **Clinique Superbalm Tinted Lip** treatment combines a sheer tint with advanced treatment benefits to lock in long-lasting shine and protection. Fresh, glossy, and moisture-rich, it provides shield and sheen when used alone or over lipstick.

• **L'Oréal Colour Riche Rich Creamy Lipcolor** provides a lasting luminous look with vitamins A and E to moisturize lips. Antifeathering formula holds a defined line and helps color stay true.

• **Dior Rouge Collection Hydrating Satin Lipstick** has a creamy texture, rich color, and leaves lips protected and moisturized.

sults if you do it yourself, but do go on to the next level of treatment if you haven't achieved the whiteness you want.

And then keep your teeth white. Whether you've had a professional bleaching or not, your teeth will need maintenance products to keep them their whitest. Now it's very simple. Following a true cosmetic approach, on-the-go whitening has become as easy as reapplying lipstick. You can whiten and brighten after lunch, a cup of coffee, a glass of wine. Two good go-anywhere options:

• GoSmile, a sleek, silver mirrored compact filled with individual, vacuum-sealed applications of 6 percent hydrogen peroxide gel. Developed by aesthetic prosthodontist Dr. Jonathan Levine, each dosage-fresh ampoule flips open, has its own little brush, and allows you to whiten up on the spot. GoSmile is sold in better specialty stores.

• The Rembrandt Whitening Wand looks like a lip gloss, and applies like one, from a sponge-tip applicator. With approximately 10 percent carbamide peroxide, it's meant to "touch-up" brightness and shine as it freshens breath. Rembrandt Oral Care products are available where you buy toothpaste.

Now you've got good reason to smile . . . your skin is glowing, your colors are right, and you've got a good feeling about yourself. It's time to go get your hair done!

# TEN

# great hair: making it modern

**How to play up gray for all it's worth— the style, the cut, the color!**

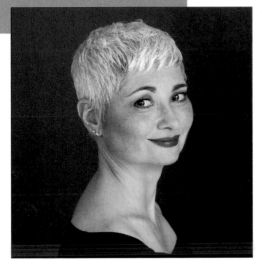

This is the moment. You've got your gray, and you want to know just how good you can look. So you call up your favorite salon and make an appointment. That's what we did, in fact, we made several appointments, with the Minardi Salon, our helpmates, guides, and gurus for the book. But now it's time to show proof of the pudding. How great can gray really be? Take a look.

We'll reveal what the stylist really said, what the colorist really thought. We'll take note of what they're wearing, too, and why. With clothes provided by Lafayette 148 New York, one of the top "bridge" lines for women in stores like Neiman Marcus and Saks Fifth Avenue, we had a fantastic range of casual-to-career-to-evening looks and a full range of sizes from which to choose. You'll see how it all comes together; the color, the style, the image. And quite possibly you'll find a look that can work for you.

### appointment: Alice Feder

The first thing to address was color. Alice had recently moved into a home supplied by well water, and her hair showed the telltale traces of green. A five-minute treatment with a clarifying shampoo helped lift out the mineral buildup, followed by ARTec White Violet Shampoo and Conditioner to tone down yellow. **The diagnosis:** Alice's hair was all one length. "Hair that just hangs there can be

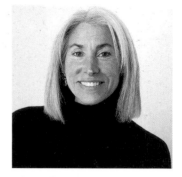

aging," advised Carmine, "and it does nothing to play up your best features. You've got great bone structure and beautiful eyes, but nothing is pointing them out." **The cut:** Layers added at the back for more fullness, with long, choppy layers around the face for a more updated look. Both of them agreed that it could be much shorter in the back. Alice said she wasn't a "bang person," but with longer pieces around the face, she can play with them—push them back or to the side one day, or bring them forward. "It just gives her more versatility," noted Carmine. Day two: Alice called to say she was thrilled with "the best haircut I ever had in my life!" **The**

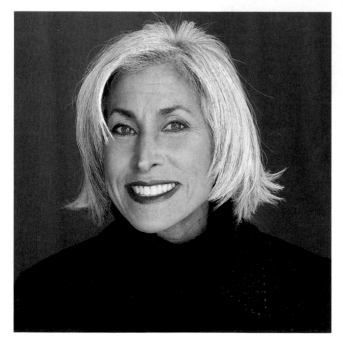

**clothes:** With a sharpened style, Alice was ready for red, in a new twist on a suit jacket from Lafayette 148. Stitch-trimmed in black, it could take a black turtleneck underneath (her favorite dressing ploy), and look polished and casual at the same time. Perfect for her job representing two radio stations: one classical and one rock. "Some days I have to look hip, some days I have to look serious," she says. "And every day, I'm a mother!"

*Hair stylist: Carmine Minardi, Minardi Salon*
*Makeup stylist: Tammy Laimos*

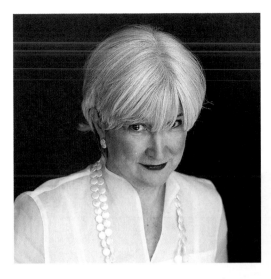

## appointment: Mia Fonssagrives Solow

Mia's midlength hair was doing nothing for her natural beauty. Because it tended to be fuller at the sides, Carmine felt it gave an "earmuff" effect. **The diagnosis:** Coarse hair, with a bit of natural curl. It needed thinning. Yet this can be tricky. "Stylists tend to get too aggressive when they thin coarse hair," says Carmine. If you cut it at midshaft, it can get wiry and stiff. When you cut too close to the roots, the hair takes over, and the cowlicks take over." **The cut:** By thinning only the last half inch of hair, with texturizing scissors, and giving the ends a bit of unevenness, Carmine kept its natural mobility. He added more layers at the back, flipping them up gently, for a more modern look. **The clothes:** Surrounded in her studio by her signature animal sculptures, Mia wears a sharply cut jacket from Lafayette 148. In fabrics like sleek silk faille, it adds a subtle touch of elegance to the equation. Mia added her own jewelry designs for artistic interest: a whimsical diamond-studded elephant necklace and "fringe" pearl earrings. Ready for her close-up, in a pristine white organza blouse with sheer yoke and sleeves, Mia proved that a sculptural style can be charmingly feminine.

*Hair stylist: Carmine Minardi, Minardi Salon*
*Makeup stylist: Jennifer Wobito*
*Jewelry: Mia Fonssagrives Solow at Gumps*

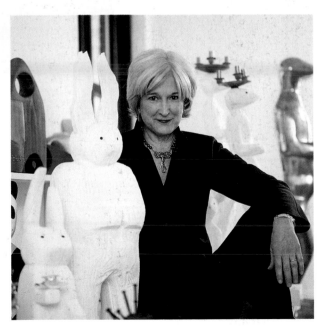

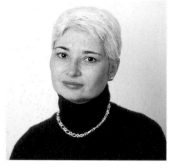

### appointment: Jo Anne Pinto

Petite and pretty, JoAnne loves a short-short style. But even the shortest look needs definition. **The diagnosis:** With gray hair, you have to make a concerted effort to keep it looking young," says Carmine, "and you can do this with lots of deliberate choppy, chunky pieces." **The cut:** More contour in back (with scalp-short hair, this accentuates and defines the shape of the head). Melanie took the bulk out of the midbottom portion, leaving a little length at the nape. "As short as it is, this makes the crown look slightly higher, makes the neck look longer, and gives her the appearance of a little more height." **The clothes:** Short hair shows off beautiful shoulders, and a ballet neckline shows off both. Lafayette 148's black jersey top has a soft drape and flare, which elevates it immediately from T-shirt status. The little touch of leather at the neckline is

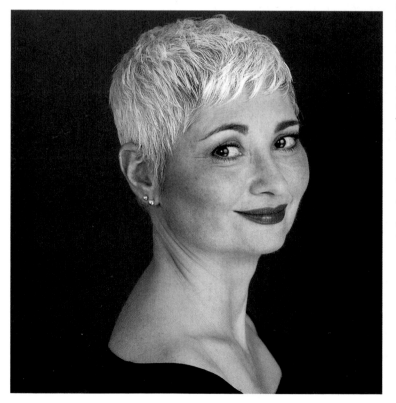

all it took to put her in black leather pants. While never wanting to imitate the clothes her nineteen-year-old daughter wears, JoAnne is a natural for a modern, young look.

*Hair stylist: Melanie Moses, Minardi Salon Makeup stylist: Jennifer Wobito*

## appointment: Rita Citrin

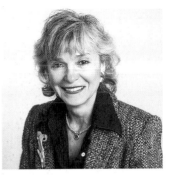

Rita's naturally wavy hair was so easy to style, she trimmed it herself. But it had a tendency to flatten out on top and was in need of a good shaping. **The diagnosis:** The overall look was doing nothing to bring out Rita's best features, and it worked against her five-three height. "When hair gets round and thick-looking, it can actually make you look shorter," advised Carmine. Heavy bangs made her face look even smaller. **The cut:** Giving her hair more lift on the top with layers solved the sinking, aided by contoured layering at the nape. "When you take the heaviness out of the midback, it acts like a corset to pop up the top." While leaving flirty wisps at the neckline, Carmine trimmed enough to elongate the neck, adding height to her appearance. Choppy, irregular bangs opened up her face and accentuated her eyes. **The clothes:** The uncluttered look was maximized by Lafayette 148's shaped, fitted

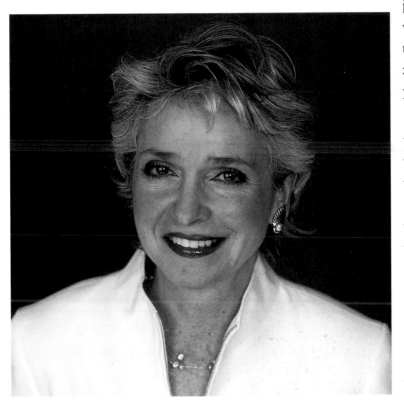

jacket in pure, pristine white. No lapels, no buttons, just a quick little zip to leave as open as you like.

*Hair stylist: Carmine Minardi, Minardi Salon*
*Makeup stylist: Jennifer Wobito*
*Necklace: Che Che New York*

**165**

### appointment: Chazz Levi

As most women do, Chazz leads multiple lives: events planner, model, wife, mom. Her hair needs to be completely adaptable, and so she wears it in the simplest style. The biggest bonus to her look: bangs! "They made my hair instantly younger-looking and sexy." **The diagnosis:** The styling products used at a recent modeling assignment had turned Chazz's hair off-color. The first thing to do was a shampoo treatment with Un-color, followed by ARTec's White Violet Conditioner. **The cut:** Melanie simply shaped up Chazz's do-it-yourself "bathroom bangs" and left her versatile blunt cut alone. **The clothes:** Never a "pastel person" pregray, Chazz has discovered the power of pure, soft color. She arrived at the shoot in pale blue head to toe, and we snapped her just the way she was!

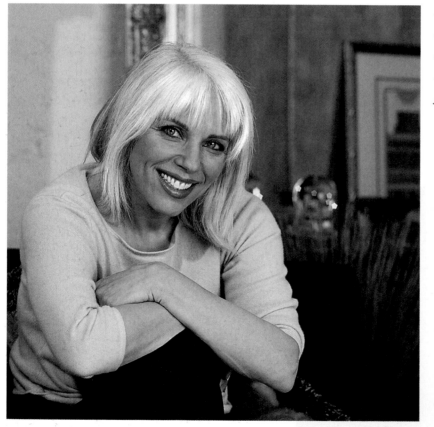

*Hair stylist: Melanie Moses, Minardi Salon Makeup stylist: Jennifer Wobito*

## appointment: Mary Louise Farrell

Mary Louise had been wearing her striking white hair pinned up at one side "forever," and wanted it to be as easy to pull back as it had always been. With hair that was all one length, she had cut short bangs at the front.

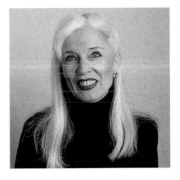

**The diagnosis:** The bangs added one little layer that didn't merge well with the straightness of the hair. Melanie felt cutting cheekbone-length layers at the side would give her the ability to pull the hair back, yet provide softness around the face. **The cut:** Mary Louise opted to keep her hair one length, with just an end trim. The softness was added with the styling. A blow-out was followed with a few rollers set diagonally on top. Brushing it out provided glamorous fullness and soft curl, super-sexy for sixty! **The clothes:** When basic black is "your color," look for ways to add light and life. Sometimes, it's built into the clothes, like Lafayette 148's matte jersey black polo with white satin collar and cuffs. A little gleam here, a little brightness there.

*Hair stylist: Melanie Moses, Minardi Salon*
*Makeup stylist: Jennifer Wobito*

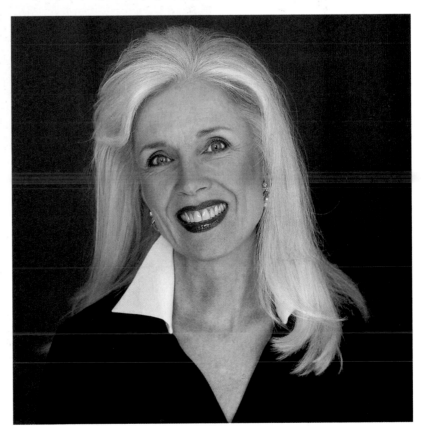

## appointment: Irene Breslaw Grapel

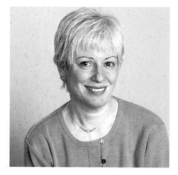

Irene's soft, silvery crop of hair had grown to an in-between length. It was in need of a good shaping, and a little updating. **The diagnosis:** Carmine focused on her bangs first. They were styled in a simple, brushed-forward look. "Bangs should never be blunt cut with gray hair," he said. "They can look artificial and wiglike." **The cut:** He cut in choppy, piecey bangs for a more modern look, and gave the hair shorter layers in back and on top to lift off the scalp. The result? A very feminine look that was younger, spikier, and much more fun. **The clothes:** Color added a complementary spark, in a rich violet shade, matched jacket to blouse. The shape was classically simple, for this classical musician, but the contrast of matte to shine added a lively note of interest.

*Hair stylist: Carmine Minardi, Minardi Salon Makeup stylist: Jennifer Wobito*

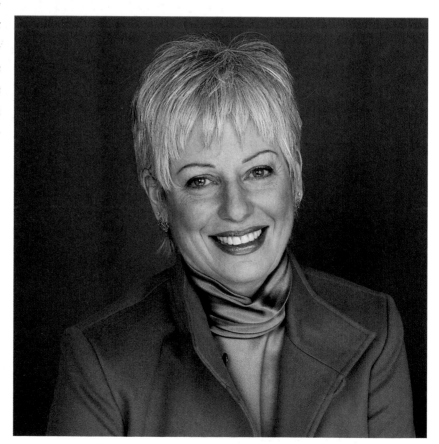

## appointment: **Setsuko Nagata Ikeda**

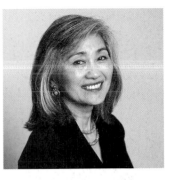

Setsuko often has to wear her hair up when she plays with the symphony, and she wanted to maintain the length. But she also wanted a bit of height. This was precisely what was needed: length without height equals roundness, the wrong shape for a round face. **The diagnosis:** Because Asian hair tends to be very straight and heavy, it needs to have movement and texture in the cut. **The cut:** Melanie lightened some of the weight by layering the crown area, giving the hair visual lift. Bringing the hair away from the face provided another lift—"an automatic face-lift," said Carmine. Finally, more layers were added in the back to lend a vertical line. **The clothes:** Pure shining silver highlighted the mélanged effect of Setsuko's hair, in Lafayette 148's simple wrap-satin shirt that can go from rehearsal hall to gala with just a switch to a long black velvet skirt.

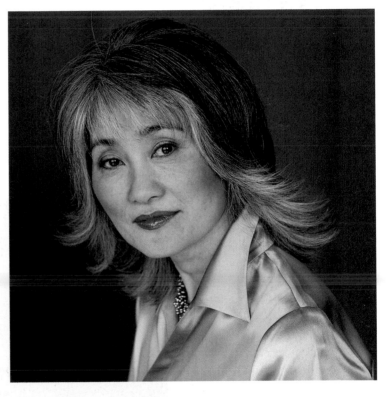

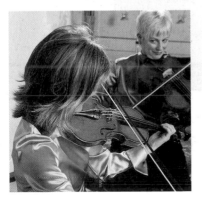

*Hair stylist: Melanie Moses, Minardi Salon*
*Makeup stylist: Jennifer Wobito*
*Jewelry: Che Che New York*

A melody of gray tones and an impromptu concert by New York Philharmonic assistant principal Viola Irene Breslaw Grapel and freelance violinist Setsuko Nagata Ikeda.

## appointment: **Amy Robinson**

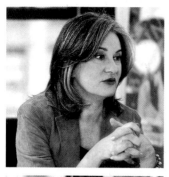

Amy's beautifully mélanged hair is just what you might ask your colorist for, if nature didn't comply. In Amy's case, it did. Soft, whiter streaks frame the face well and nicely striate the deep brunette undertone. All that's really left to do is play it all up with a cut that highlights the levels of shading. **The diagnosis:** While a longer length can get draggy, a versatile cut will give Amy the option to blow it out straight, or let it wave softly. **The cut:** Carmine cut steep angles, beginning at the cheekbone, and gave lift to the crown with medium-to-long layers. "This combination allows for volume, without being puffy," he said. "The hair will weight better in more humid conditions." A true benefit for a producer who travels the globe. **The clothes:** Seasonless versatility is key for a pack-and-go wardrobe as well. Over a go-anywhere base of black tank and pants, a lavender suede jacket adds softness and light. With details like turn-back cuffs, it gives a strong bracelet a featured role. Amy's comment: "I seem to always choose this color for photographs!"

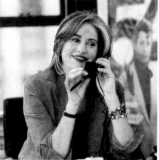

*Hair stylist: Carmine Minardi, Minardi Salon Makeup stylist: Jenn*

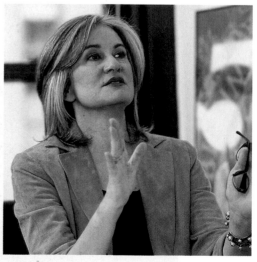

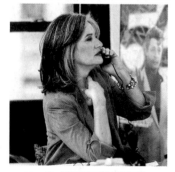

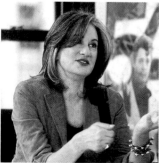

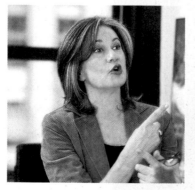

## appointment: Joan Kaner

As the fashion director of Neiman Marcus, Joan must always present a polished appearance. And her mélanged gray hair is part of it. "I never think about what color my hair is," she says. **The diagnosis:** Joan's hair has a natural wave and "goes anyway it wants to, especially the gray ones." Good shaping is vital to help it keep its chic, nonstop. **The cut:** Longer layers at the crown give short, thick hair structure and versatility. The one-length look is kept short at the sides, with slightly graduated layers in back. Joan's side-swept bangs follow a natural flow and frame the face softly. **The clothes:** Lafayette 148 moves white right into fall as ivory, in a spectacular silk/wool winter bouclé. The longer coat jacket adds textural interest to wool crepe pants and a merino turtleneck. Just the kind of polished look that can go from office to meetings to a multitude of fashion shows.

*Hair stylist: Anna Mateo, Rubann Salon Makeup stylist: Jennifer Wobito*

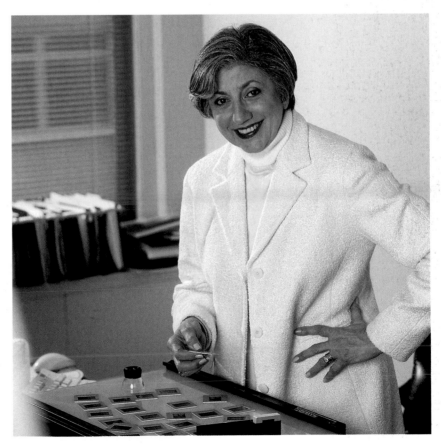

# great hair: special effects

**Sometimes gray needs a color boost. Professional techniques can enhance every strand.**

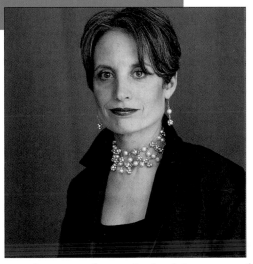

No matter what color a woman's hair is, she can look in the mirror and feel "something's missing." *What* something? That's harder to put into words. "Life," some women will say. Drama, impact, interest, contrast. You name it, if it's just not there, you know it. And, just as professional colorists can work magic on hair of any hue, they can apply the same techniques to gray hair. Not really changing the color (unless you want it changed), but simply enhancing it.

If you think in terms of your gray as a hair *color*, you'll more easily see that it opens up a whole world of possibilities. The "don't touch my gray" fear will go. Perhaps when you were blonde, you had highlights put in; maybe, as a brunette, you added a little warmth. So now you're gray, and now you think Mother Nature suddenly knows best?

It isn't the sacred shade you think—face it, it may be totally wrong for your skin tone, it may be bland and uninteresting. And it may benefit from a strategic and subtle placement of color. *Just like any hair.*

So, go ahead, find as many ways to play up your gray as you want. Investigate the techniques you see here. One of them may be all you need to go from simply gray to great!

The techniques you'll see on the following pages: highlighting, lowlighting, clarifying, glazing, and area coloring. Even though you may think you know them when you see them, let's talk about what we're talking about.

**highlighting:** Lifting color from selected strands throughout hair to create a lighter or warmer effect. Can be subtle or chunky. Involves expert placement of foils and careful timing.

**lowlighting:** Also called "reverse highlighting." Adds deeper color to selected strands to create depth and texture. Provides a subtle-to-dramatic tonal effect different from those accomplished with glazes or permanent color.

**clarifying:** The use of a special residue-removing shampoo or treatment to lift product buildup from the hair. Used to slightly lighten hair, brighten tone, or restore shine.

**glazing:** The use of a demipermanent color to add a sheer, translucent tone and lustrous shine to hair.

**area coloring:** The placement of color in predetermined sections, providing rich definition and depth. Not a "whole-head" effect; not a "selected strand" effect.

Any shade of gray, or any stage of graying, can benefit from the boost of a special color process. With gray hair that's in a transition period, a salt-and-pepper mélange, the effect will be subtle, emphasizing natural light and shadow. It can give the hair movement, energy, and depth. With pure white hair, you'll get a crisper tone, not streaks of color. The end result will be less of a flat, one-dimensional effect, far more interesting in its play of light. And, for hair that's gone dull, lifeless, and just plain blah, you'll see a sparkling, silvery difference, a refreshed, revitalized tone. It will feel like "a color" again. Talk to your salon about what may be right for you. If you're worried about starting something you may want to stop, tell them you want a procedure that leaves no obvious "grow-out" and gradually fades away. And, always remember, if you're having color work done, to treat your hair kindly and treat your hair well; healthy hair adds its own natural radiance.

# special effect: clarifying

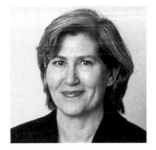

### appointment: Sherrill Adams

**The color:** New to gray, Sherrill wasn't at first convinced it was for her, and had tried semipermanent color early on. Beth Minardi got rid of all traces of that with a clarifying shampoo, then used a silverizing second shampoo to brighten and sharpen the tone. The gray, which had tended to "blend in" and dull the tone before, came to life with a clean, sparkling shine.

If there is only one thing to remember about keeping gray hair looking great, it's this: The right cut makes all the difference. Sherrill very kindly let her hair "overgrow" for this appointment, but she was desperate for a cut when the day came. **The diagnosis:** Too dense at the sides and too thick at the top. Thick hair is a luxury that lends itself well to layers, but when it gets too long, it can cause the crown to go flat, weighing the whole look down. **The cut:** Carmine kept movement in the hair by not going too short at the nape. He added more layers near the crown for lift and spiky little pieces around the face to accentuate Sherrill's great eyes. **The clothes:** Even pre-gray, Sherrill's favorite color was red, so what better choice than Lafayette 148's radiant silk dupioni red jacket, with soft jacquard waves to capture the light. Underneath, a simple black charmeuse tank top adds a bit of inner glow, and delicate strands of pearls bring more light to the face. The sharpening of line at the collar doubles the effect of a sharpened hair style. Net result: Sherrill's natural, casual style takes an elegant turn.

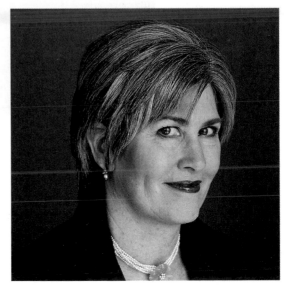

*Colorist: Beth Minardi, Minardi Salon*
*Hair stylist: Carmine Minardi,*
*Minardi Salon*
*Makeup stylist: Jennifer Wobito*
*Jewelry: Che Che New York*

# special effect: highlighting and lowlighting

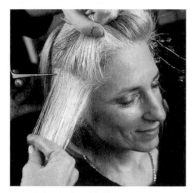

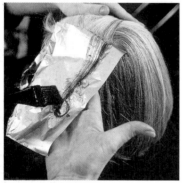

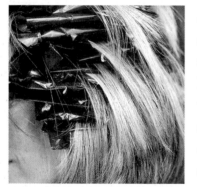

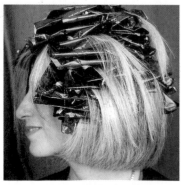

## appointment: Patricia Moscou

**The color:** Patricia, a clinical psychologist, needs to maintain a professional, no-frills appearance at all times. Yet a bit of glamour and fantasy is fun for her. Beth determined that subtle white highlights would add some "oomph" to Patricia's hair, and a few steel-like lowlights would provide body and contrast. "This is what's going to make it pop," Beth said, proving that overall color doesn't have to change to make gray hair more dramatic. "When hair is white-white, and you have icy blue eyes, that's fabulous. But when you have brown eyes, like Patricia's, it can wash you out. Her hair can be much more fun." **The diagnosis:** Too long, too straight, too do-nothing. **The cut:** Shannon updated Patricia's basic blunt cut by giving it long layers so it wouldn't flatten. "She's getting most of the volume around the bottom," Shannon noted, "and that just drops the interest too far down." With a little angling around the face, Patricia's new do was terrifically "uplifting." **The clothes:** Patricia loves dressing in gray, and this textural jacket shows just how interest-

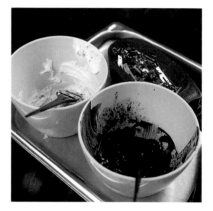

The stuff of color. A double dose for dimensional effects.

The process involves foils, and two different bowls of color; one a demipermanent silver glaze, and the other a snow-white bleach.

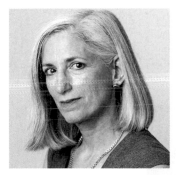

ing it can be. Lafayette 148 works a patchwork texture into a flat boiled-wool surface, softening everything with a dance of gray fur down the front. Adding this bit of romance to "serious" gray suiting delighted Patricia. "It reminds me of an ice-skater's costume!" Accessories note: The sparkle of "diamonds" can dazzle up gray, in a setting that adds a subtle metallic gleam.

*Colorist: Beth Minardi, Minardi Salon Hair stylist: Shannon Briggs, Minardi Salon Makeup stylist: Jennifer Wobito Jewelry: Mia Fonssagrives Solow at Gumps*

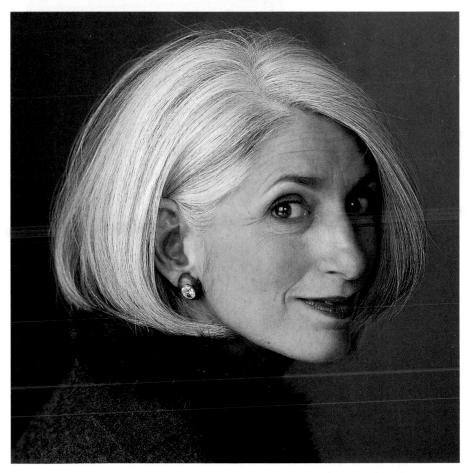

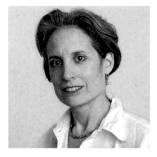

# special effect: lowlighting

### appointment: Francine Matalon-Degni

**The color:** Francine's steely shade lacked a little drama and depth. It called for a bit more "pepper" to add the spice, and that's what lowlights accomplish. Renée kept the lightness around the face, then added the darkest shade of brown by weaving and slicing, starting three-quarters back from the hairline. The process involved a demipermanent coloring, which doesn't change the structure of the hair, and ten foils going toward the bangs. "It's called back-to-back foiling," Renée said, "because you don't leave any hair out. This creates a more chunky effect." The bonus: There is no problem with grow-out lines. With a demipermanent color, the shade will gradually fade away in about two months. A final rinsing with a violet conditioner shined up the silver until it sparkled. **The diagnosis:** With hair longer than she liked, Francine had a definite "wedge" line in back. The weight of this caused the sides to be wide enough to resemble a bob. **The cut:** Carmine contoured the hair, lifting the crown with shorter layers, and reduced the diameter at the sides. The result? Hair that could be slicked back, just the way she liked to wear it, or brought forward to softly

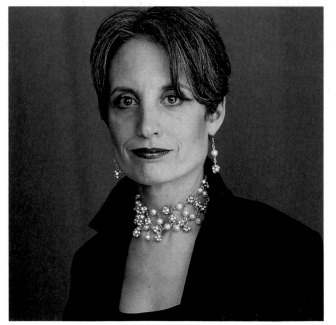

frame her face. **The clothes:** More drama was added with Lafayette 148's radiant silk dupioni jacket in a brilliant ruby shade. Tying softly in the front to add fit and shape, it is elegant enough to be worn over a taffeta evening skirt, with a bit of vintage jewelry to make the whole look glisten!

*Colorist: Renée Rockefeller, Minardi Salon*
*Hair stylist: Carmine Minardi, Minardi Salon*
*Makeup stylist: Jennifer Wobito*

# special effect: area coloring

### appointment: Amy Trakinski

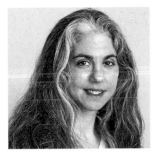

**The color:** Amy's long, naturally curly hair had started to gray the right way, with a white streak falling along a face-framing wave. But as it became more diffuse in her hair, it lost impact. **The diagnosis:** To reduce the all-over "salt" effect, Beth advised playing up Amy's natural warm undertones to take down the gray, leaving it more pronounced in the front. She combined two nonammonia products in a neutral brown and a warm brown, foiling them into selected areas. "I added 55 percent color, and left 45 percent of her hair as is," said Beth, "and this will grow out only as shadow, with no roots." She finished with an ivory white glaze treatment to add more shine and life. **The diagnosis:** Amy's natural look had become overgrown, and the weight of the hair was pulling out the natural wave in her shower-and-go style. As a young lawyer, she needed more polish. **The cut:** Carmine kept the length, eliminating only a few inches at the bottom. Then he angled it around her face, starting at the chin, in choppy layers. "This will make her hair wave better when she lets it dry naturally," he said, "and won't look too heavy when she blows it dry straight." Jennifer's expert eyebrow reshaping was the final step, and Amy's beautiful features emerged. **The clothes:** With warm beige skin tones, Amy was told she couldn't wear white. But it "popped" perfectly against her warmer shade of hair. Lafayette's mitered V-neck top combined a sexy edge with a casual attitude. Perfect for her new look.

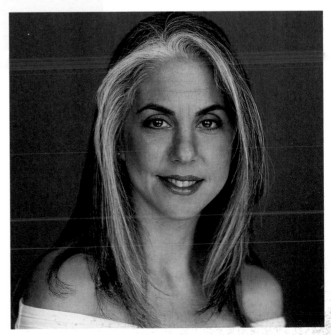

*Colorist: Beth Minardi,*
*Minardi Salon*
*Hair stylist: Carmine Minardi,*
*Minardi Salon*
*Makeup stylist: Jennifer Wobito*

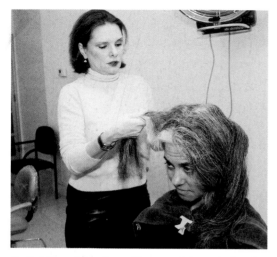

Beth Minardi begins with a careful analysis of hair texture and graying patterns.

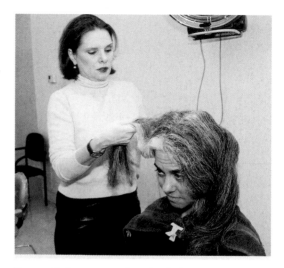

By carefully segmenting the hair, natural light is retained to frame the face.

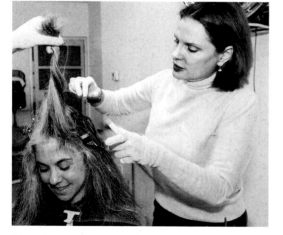

Warming up the natural undertones with area placement of color gives the deeper layers of hair added dimension.

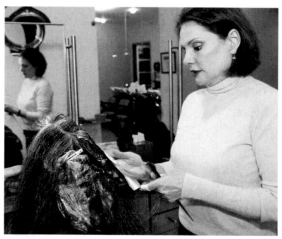

A neutral brown shade is foiled into selected areas to unify the tone.

# special effect: highs, lows and glaze

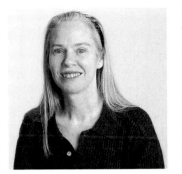

## appointment: Pat Flannery

**The color:** Pat's natural blonde had become drabbed down by the percentage of gray in her hair, and it was making her look older and too washed out. She wanted it to look more beautiful, but she didn't want high maintenance. Renée used nonammonia lowlights in back to get rid of the blahs, and added deeper areas of color in front, a quarter inch away from her hairline, averting root problems. After a few "white corn" highlights around the face to make the hair appear more baby blonde, an overall demipermanent glaze in a soft beige tone was added. "This washes out gradually and naturally within six to eight weeks," promised Renée. **The diagnosis:** Pat liked the length, so a one-inch trim was all that was necessary to revitalize the ends. **The cut:** To counteract the hair's natural limpness, Tammy sliced into the ends, adding texture and volume. She then created steep angles in the front, beginning a little below the jawline to give the hair a bit of movement around the face without adding layers. **The clothes:** The contrast of black to pale skin is always striking, and Lafayette 148's wrap-around knit top provided a sculptural neckline to play up the angles of the cut. Simple, but effective!

*Colorist: Renée Rockefeller, Minardi Salon*
*Hair stylist: Tammy Laimos, Minardi Salon*
*Makeup stylist: Jennifer Wobito*

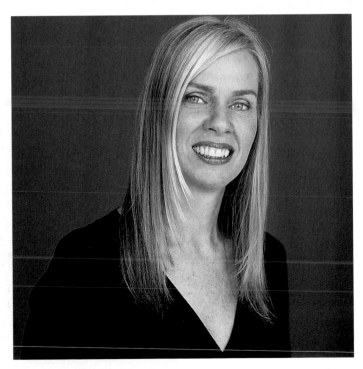

# special effect: color weaving and glazing

### appointment: Deborah Aiges

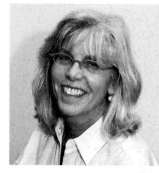

**The color:** In some lights, Deborah's hair looked silvery gray, in others, platinum blonde. In essence, it wasn't a color at all! Kenneth chose to "remember" her hair's natural sandy blonde color by foiling in two sandy shades, one slightly whiter, in chunky weaves. "This works with the existing gray," he said, "to create subtle dimensions. Yet, overall, it will have a blonde feel." With a final pearl ash blonde glaze to remove any brash tones, the hair was shining bright. **The diagnosis:** Melanie summed up the problem immediately, "Deborah has a creative job, but she doesn't have creative hair." Although she wanted it long enough to pull back when looking at layouts, it could be solved in a more interesting way. **The cut:** Melanie razor-cut the hair to introduce movement, with medium layers on top for height. She also reversed Deborah's natural left-side part, moving it to the right, for natural and immediate lift. With choppy bangs for drama, the net effect was sexier, younger, much more creative! **The clothes:** Capitalizing on a cut that pointed out Deborah's beautiful sea-blue eyes was the softness of a leather jacket and charmeuse blouse in a luminous aqua shade. The contrast of leather to shine has much the same effect as highlighting hair. You put the light where you want it. Deborah added a necklace she had made herself to go with the clothes.

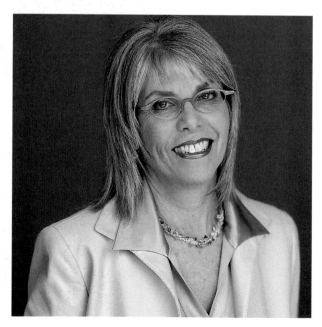

*Colorist: Kenneth Bradley,*
*Minardi Salon*
*Hair stylist: Melanie Moses,*
*Minardi Salon*
*Makeup stylist: Jennifer Wobito*
*Jewelry: Deborah Aiges*

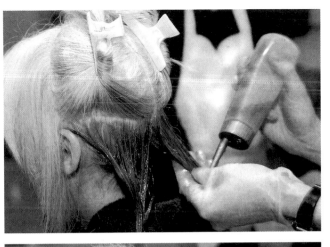

Deborah's hair is carefully sectioned, and a richer shade is added to the deeper layers.

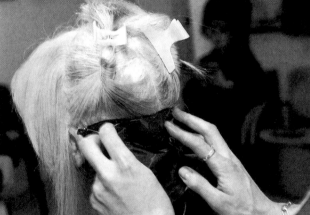

Foiled again! Toning is kept carefully segmented.

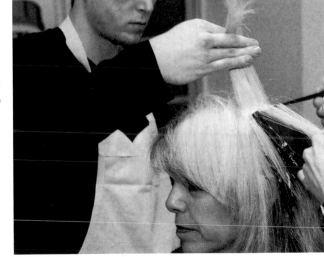

A whiter shade is added in chunky layers to create soft highlights.

increases its vulnerability. The fact that many Asians choose to perm and color their hair is risky business, indeed.

Caucasoid hair is a bit of this and a bit of that. The shaft is oval in shape. The keratin bundles are mixed; most are straight, some are wavy, accounting for the wide variety of curl and straightness. There simply is no one type; it varies widely in diameter, texture, and color. It can be coarse or fine, dense or sparse, curly or straight. Not confined exclusively to those of Caucasian heritage, Caucasoid hair covers a lot of global ground.

So don't think you have bushy Jewish hair, bouncy Spanish hair, wavy Italian hair, wooly African hair, or crinkly gypsy hair, for that matter. In the real world, if you have curly hair, you have curly hair. It doesn't matter if your ancestors crossed the Alps or the rain forest, your curly hair is unique unto itself.

"For me, there are only three kinds of hair: straight, curly, and kinky," says the acclaimed "Queen of Curl," Ouidad. "It isn't an issue of ethnicity." As the owner of a salon catering only to clients with curly, kinky, and wavy hair, Ouidad has seen curly hair of all shapes, races, and nationalities in the twenty years since she opened her salon. "I eat, walk, and talk curly hair," she says, "and I think women should celebrate it."

And so we begin this chapter with a celebration of the uniqueness of curly hair—with five crazy, wavy, hazy grays. You'll see it in all of its glory, in all of its variety, on the next pages. Following that, you'll learn why it is the way it is.

# curly girls

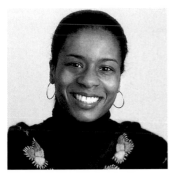

### appointment: **Dara Roche**

Although Dara loves simplicity, her thick, coarse, kinky hair requires a lot of work. And because she has had chemical straightening, the scattered strands of gray had lost some brightness. **The diagnosis:** To help restore shine and brightness, Melanie began with a violet-based shampoo. Then it was time for some advice. "Hair like this requires a lot of moisturizing, and you've got to keep the ends trimmed." **The cut:** To retain the length, Melanie suggested long layers, but not too many. "You shouldn't layer too much, because it's going to be a lot of work." Then she swept it all up in a spiky, modern style, weaving the gray into a virtual work of art! **The clothes:** The dramatic simplicity of a halter top played up the updo to the max. And, not incidentally, Dara's beautiful chinline and shoulders. Lafayette 148 provided all the decoration a look like this needs: simple shell embroidery to catch the light.

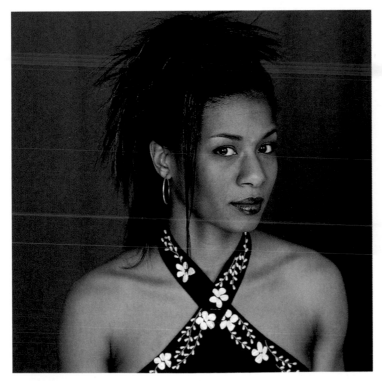

*Hair stylist: Melanie Moses, Minardi Salon Makeup stylist: Jennifer Wobito*

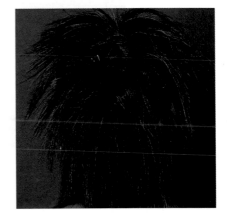

## appointment: Marilyn Sokol

As an actress, Marilyn needs maximum versatility with her hair. She never knows if a part will call for an updo, ringlets, or soft waves. If it calls for another color, however, she'll wear a wig! **The diagnosis:** No problem. Marilyn's silvery mélange and lively, bouncy curls suit her personality to a T. She helps maintain them by using Aveda's "Be Curly" cream after shampooing and in between to refresh and wake up the curl, and she always uses a shine-enhancing shampoo and conditioner. **The cut:** A recent mid-shoulder-length cut made all the difference in styling ease. "Now it's working," she said, and arrived with only a few long-neck clips in wet hair. When it dried, masses of glorious ringlets boinged up to chin length. **The clothes:** Perfect for any part, Lafayette 148's Victorian velvet "bed jacket," softly ruffled round the neck and down the front. In a rich burgundy shade, it played up Marilyn's coloring to great applause!

*Hair stylist: Carsten of Carsten Union Square, NYC Makeup stylist: Jennifer Wobito*

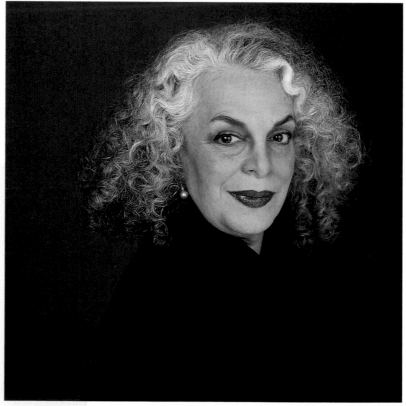

## appointment: Jennie Benard

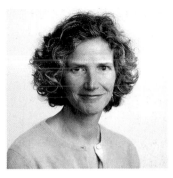

Jennie's naturally wavy hair provides a delicate, doll-like frame for her fine features. A natural blonde who never colored her hair, she likes the multitude of new tones that graying has added. **The diagnosis:** Because Jennie's hair tends to frizz when she attempts to brush the curls out, a let-it-wave style works best. **The cut:** Sachi reduced bulk through the nape, bringing the curls a little closer to the neck. She kept the sides layered, building in levels that would lighten the weight of its length. **The clothes:** To offset any "busy-ness" that curls can add to a look, pure lines and pure color work best. We chose the uncluttered, sophisticated look of Lafayette 148's gleaming white charmeuse shirt.

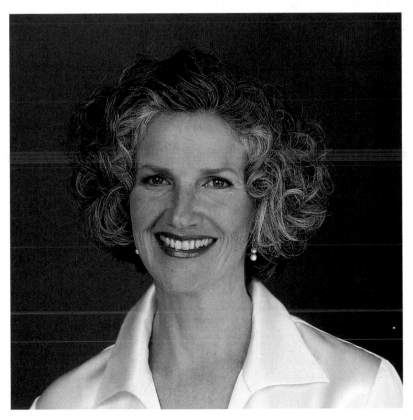

*Hair stylist: Sachi Fukumoto, Minardi Salon Makeup stylist: Jennifer Wobito*

### appointment: Carmine Fuentes

Carmine has been celebrating both her natural curls and her sensational white-gray for almost the same number of years; thirty for the curls, twenty-five for gray, and fifteen since her curls have "really been out there." **The diagnosis:** Because she has an "utter frizz ball" if she shampoos too often, Carmine relies on a good conditioner, a climate control defrizzer, and a botanical spray, all Ouidad products, to keep curls fresh and in manageable condition between shampoos. **The cut:** A recent cut at the Ouidad salon reduced the weight of her almost waist-length hair, and gave Carmine's curls more bounce and life. "Now that it has a good cut," she says, "I can manage it pretty well by myself." **The clothes:** Although her daily look is most likely surgical scrubs, Carmine brings touches of femininity to everything she wears. Underscoring a strict lab jacket here, rich color, embroidery details, and the dash of pretty jewelry. All her own.

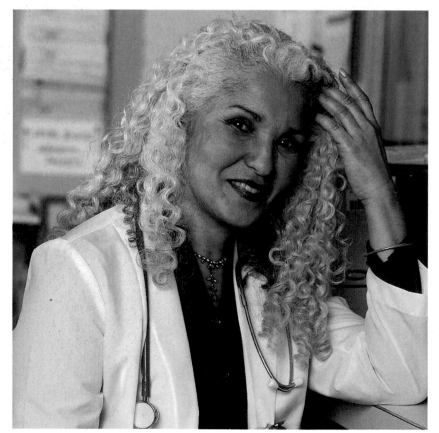

*Hair stylist: Ayanna Augustine, Ouidad Salon Makeup stylist: Jennifer Wobito*

## appointment: Ruth Lawson

Actually, no appointment was needed for Ruth Lawson; the intricate braids she keeps in her hair tames its natural, kinky fullness, and were precisely what we wanted to show. Like strands of pure, woven sterling, the color took on an amazing texture. Yet, all was pliable enough to style as she liked. Ruth only admitted to one problem: "It's hard to find artificial hair in gray for the extensions." She had; and it was woven in from the roots so inconspicuously, you never knew where her natural hair left off and the

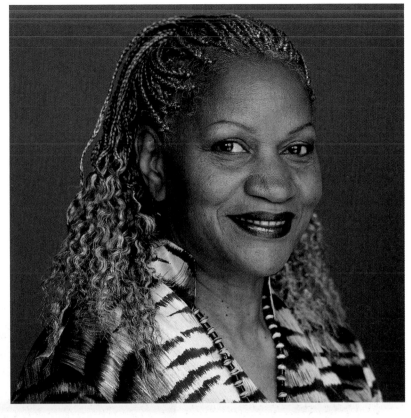

extensions took over. **The clothes:** Ruth prefers loose-fitting layers, but proved a shaped wrap blouse can define a fuller figure beautifully. Lafayette 148's sexy tiger-striped print played up her skin tone and added a completely untamed flair!

*Makeup stylist: Jennifer Wobito*

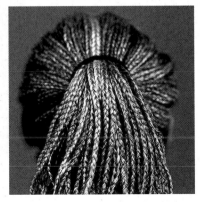

## so what's the problem? "When you have gorgeous silver curls, that is your crown," says Ouidad. "The dimension of light just bounces off it."

## "It's like looking at diamonds; it sparkles."

But what if it doesn't? Why can curly, bouncy hair look wonderful on little girls, fascinating on young women, and, if not treated well, just plain dowdy when hair turns gray? It's a matter of hair health. Light can be trapped in its webs and shadows, as can oils, grease and environmental grime. Curly hair can be starved for moisture, and that's when it turns to frizz.

## hazy gray frizz If your curly hair is gray, dry, and frizzy—it can look more like a mat than anything else. It's going to look colorless and old. Not sterling, not platinum, not even a striking mélange. Just colorless. Clueless. If you allow frizz to infiltrate your gray, you're missing something.

> "There's absolutely no excuse for unhealthy-looking hair, no matter what your style is about."
> *Carmine Minardi*

Admittedly, there are women who like the individuality of big, wooly, fuzzy hair. They use it as an art statement, a bohemian statement, a cultural statement. And that, of course, is a personal option. *But.* "At least they should put some kind of topical shiner on the hair," advises Carmine Minardi, "an oil, a silicone, a leave-in type of conditioner. If you're going to make it funky, make it funky-right."

Ouidad is the first to admit that treatments are merely a supplement to treating your whole body well. "Everyone wants miracle products," she says. "I tell women, 'You are the miracle!' We have to look at things from the inside out. We're a cosmetic society, but that's not really helping the situation. Why not eat properly, get enough sleep, get enough exercise? Fix it from the inside, and have hair that's permanently shiny and healthy."

Nourishment is the key, but so is gentle care. Curly hair puts up a strong front, especially if you have masses of it, but it's really weaker to begin with. Curly or kinky hair requires periodic replenishing of protein and moisture to maintain its healthy luster and shine. Conditioning quenches the thirst of the hair; leave-in conditioners seal in moisture. And deep, nourishing treatments, at least once or twice a month, are absolutely essential. Remember what we said about "feeding your head" in chapter five? Hair is composed of protein, likes protein, needs protein. If it's frizzy and fat, it's really starving to death.

## Frizz IZ:

- A disconnection of internal hair molecules due to dehydration
- A loss of weight in the inner layer of the hair
- A spongelike condition of the cuticle
- A bulging of the hair shaft, causing hair to lift
- Dry-looking, dull-looking, and defiant

## Frizz IZn't:

- An extreme state of curl
- Something that happens only when it rains
- A condition known only to those with natural curl in their hair
- Something you can't do anything about

> "Frizz is your hair's way of saying it's thirsty, it is not a natural quality of the hair. Your hair is hungry and thirsty. Feed it, and you'll see it perform for you."
> *Ouidad, founder, Ouidad Salon*

**kinky frizz, a double whammy** Now, if your cuticle is already "lifted" away from the shaft, as it is with curly or kinky hair, it's like a welcome sign to frizz. When the cuticle is jagged, or has sharply kinked edges, it's going to let humidity in, and vital protein molecules and amino acids out. The disconnected infrastructure has less strength, less substance. So it sucks humidity in like a straw, plumps up, pops up . . . and *frizzes*. It's only doing it because it wants a drink. But moisture without some kind of sealant isn't any good. You can't just spritz water on hair and expect it to stay in the shaft. It evaporates. That's why you need treatments and conditioners. They act to fill in the spaces, close the cuticle, and make it water-tight.

Ouidad explains, "To have light reflect off of hair, it has to be internally connected and have its own weight. Hair that's separated from itself loses that, and that's when it tends to dry and get frizzy. You have to reconnect the molecular layer, and let its own pulse beat."

And what about a bit of antifrizz treatment to tame the ones that refuse to stay straight? Some women with a structural kink to their hair simply give up on them. "If my hair's going to frizz, it's going to frizz. My hair always wins," says Dara Roche, a producer with CBS morning news.

You can't fight frizz with fire—but you can with moisture. Ouidad's Climate Control Heat & Humidity Gel, winner of the "best defrizzer" award from *Allure* magazine, doesn't attempt to slick wayward strands down. It actually grabs moisture from the air, to hydrate each strand and give frizz what it's crying out for.

**earth, wind and fire** You may have liked the band, but your hair wants nothing to do with any of these elements. Environmental pollution can build up on the scalp and the hair, blocking hair follicles from receiving vital nutrients. Air blows an ill wind, whether it's nature's own, electric heating, or air-conditioning, robbing hair of moisture. And fire, in the form of hot blow-dryers, can parch hair even more, and can actually singe the ends. Curly hair, in fact, should avoid the highest settings altogether.

There's one more evil element to add to the list: water. How come, if your hair needs an abundance of moisture? When you shampoo with warm water, the cuticle opens up even more to let cleansing agents in. It's a two-way street, again. Nutrients flow out with the shower water, and the hair is left parched and depleted. Just like your skin is when you wash your face.

So think your curls can't live in the real world? Enemies everywhere? Sure they can. But you simply have to learn how to give back what nature takes away.

## the answer, my friend, may not be blowin' in the wind. You know that definition is what gives curl shine, shape, dimension. It's really all architecture. If your locks are left untended, to blow where they want to blow, your hair loses a sense of cohesiveness, and with it, the shine and structure.

There are a variety of ways to give curly and kinky hair some structure. Sometimes you can accomplish it with your setting, or your styling. Sometimes it has to do with your cut. Ouidad invented, and is teaching to salons around the country, a method of cutting hair she calls "carving and slicing," a way of cutting *with* the wave of the curl, so each curl cups gracefully into another one, rather than stacking on top, which can be flattening. "You should never thin, layer, or 'texturize' curly hair," she advises. According to the curl expert, layering creates levels that can curl up into fat rolls. Thinning creates a mix of short and long hair that can shrink up on the short side and limp out on the long side. And "texturizing," which involves snipping random pieces of hair, can unbalance waves and send them straight into frizz.

If you set your curls, there are ways to do it that encourage definition as well. Carmine Minardi advises the use of rollers, pin curls, or a curling iron. These methods compress the cuticle and make it look like curl, not like frizz. They give definition to the curl.

Styling is another story. Many stories. Sure, you can blow it straight. But the richest, most inventive styling traditions come from cultures with more kink in their hair than curl.

## let's twist again? If the cuticle is sharply kinked, it is particularly vulnerable to all forms of physical and chemical abuse. Yes, that means chemical relaxing and coloring, but hair also suffers from the stress of tight braiding. "Mini braids break the daylights out of your hair," says Ouidad. "They're very damaging. I tell women to just cut them off and let the hair go. They say okay. *Okay?* What does that tell you?"

The complexities of braiding, weaving, and twisting kinky hair can be just as injurious as forcing it to go straight. Multiple braids have weight, extensions add more, and beads even more. Suddenly, women find their hairlines receding, and their hair breaking off.

In addition, there are other dangers lurking behind weaves, braids, and extensions. Buying the wrong kind of hair can present a problem. Synthetic hair can cause allergic reactions, even scalp conditions like eczema or seborrhea. The glue used may cause a hair-loss situation that can escalate over the months. You must always seek out quality raw hair, and then maintain your braids with washing, conditioning, and retightening every two weeks.

Maintaining hair that is twisted or braided takes special care to keep both hair and scalp healthy. A million tiny braids can be washed just as they are, without unbraiding. "I always tell people it's like you have a knitted sweater," says Lanell Goodman, a California artist who once had over four hundred braids in her hair. "Think of hair as the yarn, and the braid as the knitted stitch. You don't unravel a sweater to wash it. You don't unravel a braid, either."

If cleansing is an easy matter, conditioning the scalp isn't. "You have to get in there and oil that scalp so it doesn't become dry," says Ruth Robinson, a publishing house office manager, "and that's very time consuming." At the same time, she cautions against putting too much oil on the hair itself—it can get slippery, reducing the very traction that holds braided-twisted-wrappy styles together.

Lanell Goodman treated her micros with extra care, occasionally giving her hair a hot oil/hot towel treatment to condition the scalp, especially after braiding. "The scalp is under a lot of stress after braiding is done," she says. "It can be itchy at the beginning, it can be headachy for a couple of days. Some girls can't do this; their scalp is too sensitive and the headaches don't go away."

But then she cut. Cut them all off, to save both hair and scalp. "Every once in a while, you've got to prune," she admits. "Just clip them back, and let the scalp breathe."

There are always exceptions. Ruth Lawson, the workshop leader and trainer you first met in chapter four, has never had a day's problem with her sterling braids, and it could be because they're just a bit thicker, definitely not micro. "It's a great way to do your hair if you don't want to do anything to it," she says. "I just shampoo and that's it. No conditioner or anything. I think it shines." So how come? It could be because she gets it braided only "every so often."

**an open-and-shut case** When twists are left in the hair for a long time, they will lock. Or they can be made to lock by teasing the hair into a knotty, ropelike twist. Finer hair may be matted with a substance like beeswax to create a fused effect. But whatever the method, hair eventually acts like "whole cloth." And that's when dreads lose their life. The hair can't breathe, the scalp can't breathe, and no comb on earth is going to distribute oil down the shaft, so dreads have a signature dusty, dry look. While locking is the antithesis of hair health, many see it as a celebration of culture and pride.

But even dreads can be given a certain amount of structure and shine. Each piece may be individually gelled and twisted, then gathered together in a loose ponytail at the nape of the neck. Or, occasionally, a dab of pomade may be applied.

**natural inclinations** Ruth Lawson considers her braids "going natural," in the sense that she never subjects them to chemicals or heat. But she once let her full halo of kinky hair go its own way, in an Afro style. "That really requires maintenance and care," she says. "The only time it doesn't is if it's very close to the scalp, almost bald. Otherwise, you have to wash it and keep a conditioner on it. And you have to pick it constantly to keep it shaped and smooth. Every morning, when you wake up, it's bent out of shape. It takes a lot of work."

But even a scalp-short cut takes a certain amount of tender care. Ruth Robinson, with her micronatural, is meticulous about shine and control. She uses a pomade daily, brushes it "a lot," and adds a touch of gel on top to keep her less-than-eyelash-length hair in place. "I notice every little hair," she says, "so I like it slicked down as much as possible."

Scalp and hair health is the number-one priority for women with short, kinked hair. And most of the ones I spoke to use a combination of treatments. Janice Bryant, copy editor for *Essence* magazine, shampoos and conditions her micronatural every day. Then she uses a little freesia oil on it. "It's light, and I like the smell," she says, "like aromatherapy for the hair."

"My hair stays pretty healthy in a natural state," says Lanell Goodman, who pruned her microbraids into a clipped crop. "I'm not curling it or blow-drying it, and I really kind of like the freedom.

> "I've been through all the hair things—I've been hair and back—and I find the easiest way to look the most attractive and be the most comfortable is what you should do."

**let it go, let it flow** So you want to let your natural style live large? Be prepared for it to look grayer. When light shines through the hair, the gray stands out. "I didn't know I had that much gray," says Dara Roche, who wears her coal-colored hair midlength and straight.

> "But once when I wore it curly, a friend told me I looked like I had cobwebs in my hair."

Joan Parks, who works for a publishing house, had a similar reaction. "I did wear it natural for two summers," she says, "but when the sun hit my hair it made the color look lighter, and then I also had the gray, so I looked like a seeding dandelion. It was weird." Today Joan wears her hair midlength, and uses a "special hair relaxer." But she sticks to a strict regimen of conditioning. "I use a shampoo with a conditioner in it, and then I condition again with a leave-in moisturizer. Then I use shea butter as a daily conditioner to add gloss. Every other week I use a cholesterol treatment. I probably do too much," she confesses.

Maybe not.

Carmine Fuentes lets her long, curly hair flow free, but she pays the same kind of attention to conditioning because it can look a little dull. "I always condition when I wash it, always," she says, "but I also use a little conditioner in between shampoos, especially if it's humid out. Then I might also add a botanical spray and a climate control product if I need it." As an RN in obstetrics and a certified lactation consultant, Carmine has a hectic schedule. But caring for her curls doesn't take much time at all. Following a shampoo, she uses a combination of diffuser to "really hold the curl" and air-drying, and that's it.

**playing it straight** Chemical relaxers are potent; there's no doubt about it. Sodium hydroxide, in solutions normally ranging from 11 to 13 percent, can lift the curl and the kink out of hair, but they can also lift the life right out of it. Or worse, cause it to snap when stretched. As can any other chemical process designed to make hair do what it wasn't born to, if it's particularly vulnerable. Since curly, kinky, or gray hair is naturally weaker, put them all together, and you've got to be careful.

"I used to use chemical relaxers," says Ruth Robinson, "and I would dye my hair at the same time. I did it two weeks apart, but by the time I got done with one thing, it was time to do the other. It got to be too much, and my hair started breaking off." Then she cut it scalp-short and skipped the dye, and she admits, "I like it better."

The application of heat is another way to straighten hair, either through blow-drying or using a flat iron. Anything you use or do that makes the hair dry has to be handled carefully. Yes, you can use heat to create a straighter look, but use diffuser attachments simply to soften the curl, or lower settings on your blow-dryer if you're going after a straighter look. Don't blast away at it, and don't tug down hard. Leave a little conditioner on the ends of your hair before you hit it with heat. Deep condition regularly. And avoid doing this every day. Let your curls loose, and let them live.

When extremely curly hair is flattened, it becomes weak and dry. You may be doing it to increase the shine, but if the hair goes dry on you, it gets dull. You'll need to add moisture, and take extra precaution against heat damage, with oils, humectants, and rich, creamy conditioners. If you're going to use styling aids like gels or mousses, choose them carefully. They can get caught in a web of dry, frizzy hair, and look like little pieces of glue. A pomade, with very little wax in it, may be your best bet.

Of course, not overtaxing the hair to begin with may be the best defense against its natural vulnerability. "My hair is as close to natural as you can get," says Dara Roche. "Relaxing and chemicals can ruin your hair, and then you have to use more products to make up for it. It just doesn't make sense.

> "Leaving it alone is better, health-wise.
> There's nothing better than that."

**why is asian hair like curly hair?** For starters, sometimes it is curly. Chinese-born Marilyn Ko, an entrepreneurial forty-year-old, says her hair has been naturally wavy from birth. It is typically porous; it fattens and frizzes with high humidity, and even "absorbs cooking odors like a sponge." Marilyn did resort to chemically straightening it, "once," a complete antithesis to the overperming that causes the most amount of damage to Asian hair.

If you've got jagged, kinky cuticles, you've probably looked at silky-straight Asian hair with a mild degree of envy. You can stop. Chemically compromised or not, porous Asian hair has a similar spongelike quality. And it takes quite the same kind of special care. The most gentle shampoos, those with a lower pH level (5.0 to 5.5), are recommended, especially if you wash your hair every day. Conditioner? Absolutely. Choose a creamy one that doesn't weigh hair down; avoid those that contain silicones. An occasional penetrating conditioning treatment, like a protein pack, is a good idea to restore shine, smoothness, and vitality. Marilyn Ko uses "plain supermarket olive oil" to do the trick. Once a week, she gives her hair a half-hour conditioning with olive oil for shine and nutrition. "I've tried other oils, sesame oil and a vegetable oil, but they weigh the hair down and flatten it."

**east is east, but it isn't gray** Although Marilyn claims the pace of constant global travel and operating both a Chinese antiques store and a fashion handbag shop in New York is "making her gray," the secretive strands are hidden underneath the lustrous, dark top layers of hair. In spite of this, she does color her hair, and that's not surprising.

Gray hair is an anathema to most Asian women. A younger generation is now switching over to shades of blonde and red, in an edgy break with tradition, but deep black is still the color of choice among women who have a right to be gray. So what is it about Eastern women that causes them to cling to color? Isn't this a society that respects its elders? "That's a different story," laughs Marilyn. "We respect the wisdom and life experience of age, but not the look!"

"By fifty, Asian women are gray, no matter what they do to it," Setsuko Nagata Ikeda tells us. One of the few who allow lovely streaks of white to infiltrate her hair, Setsuko did the expected thing: she had it colored professionally for a short time. But she felt guilty about it. "When people complimented me, I felt, it's not me. Now I feel so much better; it's not my dye color they're complimenting, it's all me!"

Still, she copes with a certain shock factor when she returns to Japan. "When I go to Beijing on tour with the Philharmonic," says the violinist, people stop on the street and stare at me. Every one of them. It's like they've never seen anything like it before.

## "I get compliments in America all the time, but in Asia, they think I'm crazy."

Fortunately, Setsuko's husband, also a musician, and also gray, does not. "He tells me it's a relief to see me when we're in Japan, because everyone else is in color."

There is one advantage to being a salt-and-pepper Asian. Maintaining a bright, silvery shade of gray doesn't seem to be a problem. Setsuko says she never notices a yellow cast to her gray, and doesn't use any of those "blue shampoos." If you'll remember your color tonality lesson from chapter three, black hair has the maximum amount of blue molecules in it. It's like having a built-in blue shampoo! You can see how pretty Setsuko's hair looks in chapter ten.

## hispanic hair: all of the above
You know now there is no such thing as Hispanic hair. Like all Caucasoid hair, it may be coarse, wavy, or curly. It may be heavy and straight, but tend to become unruly in high humidity. It may be a multiethnic blend and have some kink in the structure. And it can become dry, lifeless, unmanageable, and frizzy. Just like all the hair in the world.

Dealing with all the waves and whims of curly hair has already been covered in this chapter. And products for it are recommended in chapter six. Products that weightlessly tame and smooth the cuticle; moisturize and lusterize the hair; provide volume reduction, curl definition, and some amount of discipline may be for you.

## hispanic attitude: a different story
So that leaves us only one thing to talk about here. Attitude. There *is* a cultural difference in the way gray hair is perceived and accepted. Just as Asians tend to avoid it, women of Latin heritage embrace it. At least in some countries.

Silvia Maginnis, a United Nations interpreter who hails from Argentina, never minded going gray. "I really went gray in my teens, enough for people to identify me as the tall girl with gray hair. But my mother had gray hair and was always getting compliments, so I never associated it with anything bad."

Today, as chief of the Spanish section for the General Assembly, Silvia maintains a chic, simple look. Her father, in the "rag business," gave her a lesson she lives by. "He told me, 'You have to know what looks good on you.' And so I learned, at a very young age." Part of her look is her striking white hair, and she is very comfortable with it. "Gray hair in Argentina is always considered to be very distinguished, very soignée. But Latina women project a lot of femininity, no matter what their age, so being gray does not become an issue."

Indeed, Latin style dramatizes the whole progress of a woman's life. It doesn't single out "youth" as the equivalent of beauty. While it can be a highly dynamic style, it is a pure expression of ageless, glorious, female power.

And, indeed, men of Spanish heritage are duly appreciative. More than "not minding" when a woman turns gray, many find it quite appealing. (See Man Meter on the following pages.) The fascination with gray may apply to men from Mediterranean countries as well. Italian-born photographer Andrea Morini sums up his feelings this way, "That color hair is so noble; it's super. I've always liked women with gray hair. It's intriguing." Aha! Can we suspect a hot-climate proclivity to the icy cool of gray?

Amateur anthropology notwithstanding, Silvia Maginnis offers as good an explanation as any for this phenomenon. "We've trained them." She smiles. "Women in our countries don't go in for the extreme casualness of Americans. An older

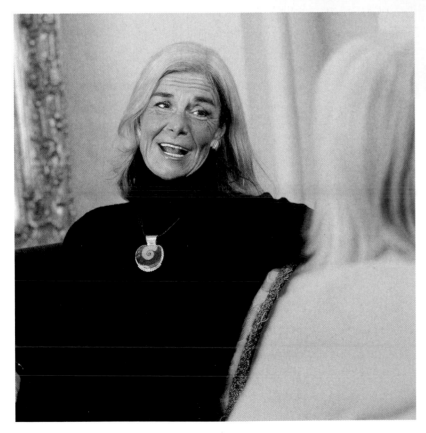

woman with gray hair is very pulled together; she's an attractive, seductive woman, and Latin men are used to noticing."

A lesson for us all.

Silvia Maginnis
*Makeup:* Jennifer Wobito
*Jewelry:* Georgina
Saccone for Southern
Artisans

# man meter

I heard it far too often to ignore. From the very first panel discussion to the very last interview, women with less color in their hair said men with more color in their skin were crazy for gray! It attracted them like a magnet. And the younger they were, the more they liked it.

"What is it with Spanish men? They come up to me all the time and comment on my hair. I get, 'Ohhh, mamacita,' when I walk down the street. I think they must have a mother complex."

*Mia Fonssagrives Solow*

"I find ethnic men come up to me very often, young men, they think it's so cool. It's a little racy. They love it. White men don't like my hair too much. It scares them."

*Peri Wolfman*

"It happens to me all the time. I mean, I meet other men, but it's always the Spanish guys who say something."

*Ellen Fox*

"I normally don't get compliments from other, nonethnic men. They don't really want to talk about it."

*JoAnne Pinto*

"Maybe it's more natural that men of color compliment my hair, but it's true. If white men compliment me, it's not about my hair."
*Angela Muriel*

"I am constantly being stopped by young people; they think it's sensational. Especially men of color and Latinos."
*Joan Kaner*

"When my braids were salt and pepper, men in their late twenties started coming on to me."
*Lanell Goodman*

"The old men never say anything to me, but the young men rush me."
*Ruth Lawson*

"Young guys like it. They stop me on the street all the time and say, 'Your hair looks so good—what is that—do you have dye on it?' "
*Janice Bryant*

# THIRTEEN
# who's great at being gray?

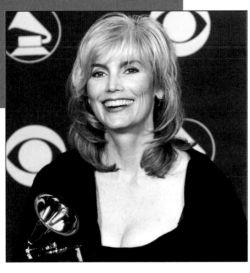

**There's a whole new "cool" to gray. Works for celebrities, men, models.**

Emmylou Harris wins awards for singing . . . and for the confidence to be gray, young-looking, and great!
© Reuters NewMedia Inc./CORBIS

You'd think people in the public eye would shun gray as they do double chins. Not so. Some actually get better-looking as they get grayer (think Richard Gere, Harrison Ford). But those are men, you say. True. The "silver" screen has been decidedly antisilver for women, until recently. But now women in the spotlight are beginning—just beginning—to be unabashedly unafraid of going gray right before your eyes: Emmylou Harris, Rita Moreno, Nancy Wilson, and Tyne Daly are among the few gray blazers.

But, in the entertainment fields, there's still a wide gulf between the sultry platinum blondes and the silvery platinum grays, and anything that even smacks of aging is hazardous to careers.

"It's hard for women actresses over thirty-five anyway," says Amy Robinson, who has produced numerous feature films, including *For Love of the Game, Autumn in New York, Never Again, From Hell, White Palace, Once Around, Chilly Scenes of Winter,* and *Running on Empty.* "Leading men who are older want leading women twenty years younger; that's the way it is. This industry is so oriented to youth and appearance that I don't see many [women stars] going gray on their own. They'll go gray for a part, or any color for that matter, but it's the part that determines hair color. And it will be that way until there's an incredibly sexy role written and the woman who plays it just happens to have silver-gray hair. It would take someone who's really out there, but I don't know when we'll see it."

### gray rocks when it comes off

Of course, gray is a statement easily made among the young and famous. Rockers "go platinum" or pure white before switching off to another shade. A few years ago, silver was all the rage among young models in Paris. And chunky hunks of bright white can show up as often as pink (or green) among the young. Gray wanna-bes are part of modern pop culture. But even "real" grays indulge in a touch of fantasy. "I saw a woman the other day, an older woman, with a pure gray kind of Afro," says Amy Robinson, "and she had put a green streak in it. Like the kids. This was her statement. I smiled at her, and she smiled back, gray to gray. It's kind of like a sisterhood."

### this just in

So why do TV anchormen get away with gray? Maybe Walter Cronkite started the "senior statesman of news" look, but ever since, others have gone well into silver territory, and even younger correspondents and field reporters have been showing a little more salt in recent years. It's the credibility thing. Older and wiser applies if you're a man. But is gray making headlines with women anchors?

"Never going to happen," predicts Licia Hahn, stylist consultant to many anchors and reporters at Fox Television. "The news is all about entertainment, and so the on-air talent is competing with Hollywood celebrities. Some of the stations have actually hired celebrities as news anchors. So a young, attractive appearance is an important asset for a serious newswoman. Television is still all about youth, sex, and ratings."

It seems the prevailing thinking on the big and small screen is that gray isn't sexy. But go to the theater, go to a cabaret. Stage performers consistently prove that it is.

**curtain calls** Broadway star Louise Pitre, who's wowed audiences coast to coast and in Canada in the hit play *Mamma Mia!*, tosses her sexy silver locks with abandon on stage. Winning almost every theater award that it's possible to win for her high-voltage portrayal of single-mother Donna Sheridan in the ABBA-inspired musical, the Canadian-born actress and singer has a successful concert and recording career as well. Always in the spotlight, she's made gray hair sexy, powerful, and beautiful.

Jamie deRoy, award-winning cabaret artist and producer-host of her own weekly television variety show, *Jamie deRoy & Friends*, has a booming career as well, in spite of the fact that she first became known as "the girl with the gray hair." She's done guest spots on numerous television series, has appeared in feature films like *GoodFellas*

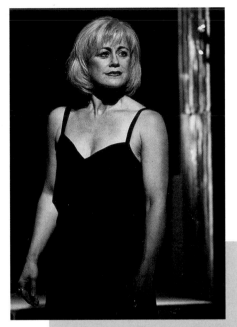

Louise Pitre in *Mamma Mia!*
Silver and sensational.
© Joan Marcus

and *Raging Bull,* and has headlined at most major clubs in New York and Los Angeles. The effervescent singer/comedienne also produces CDs, Emmy Award–winning series, and songwriter showcases, all while being gloriously silver-haired.

**you'll never work in this town** "It became my trademark," she says. "At first, everybody would tell me, 'You're never gonna get a job with gray hair,' so I put henna on it, and then a semipermanent color, and it looked like I had an extensive streak job. But people never stopped me anymore to tell me how fabulous my hair was." As strange luck would have it, there were professional disadvantages as well. "Literally, the minute after I dyed my hair, I got a call to go up for a Grecian Formula commercial. Then I had to call around to find

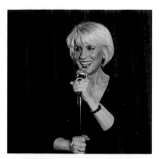

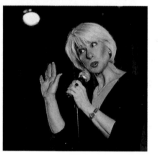

out how to get the color out, but it really didn't come out very well. So I didn't get the job. Who knows if the reason was really my hair, but I never wanted to color it again after that. This was going to be it—I was never going to touch it again." And she didn't.

When Jamie went west, to the land of the platinum blondes, she ran into the same story. A Hollywood manager insisted she color her hair. "I told him, 'The one thing I've found is that everybody remembers me because of my hair.' I figured I didn't have the same looks as everybody in L.A., or the same figure, so that was okay—I'll be the girl with the silver hair."

Today, with her striking white hair, the vivacious cabaret star looks young, sexy, and vibrant. "I've always been a natural person—I wanted to be me. And the lighter it got, the more I liked it. Now I love it."

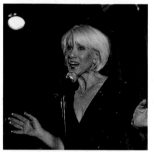

As a cabaret entertainer, Jamie needs hair that lights up under lights, and lasts till the wee small hours of the morning. It must have movement and flair, without being stiff and "set-looking."

**The diagnosis:** Jamie's hair has a lot of weight, and the thick bangs were upstaging her face. **The cut:** Tammy graduated the nape to add height at the crown, then concentrated on making the ends less bulky. By angling the sides, she eliminated the "matronly" effect caused by the sides tending to curl under. Finally—the bangs were in for a bit of texturizing to make the pieces thinner and give her overall look more of a modern edge. **The clothes:** On stage, Jamie likes to give 'em the old razzle-dazzle, in Lafayette 148's low V-neck top, studded with light-reflecting beads.

*Hair stylist: Tammy Laimos*
*Makeup stylist: Jennifer Wobito*

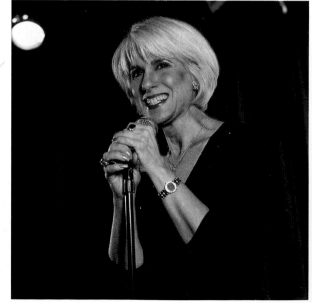

**male call** Who's also great at being gray? Men. Or at least we think so. "We see men as better-looking as they get older," says Amy Robinson, "but that's because we are culturally attuned to it. Gray hair means admitting to a certain age, and for men, that's okay."

The truth of the matter is, they're much better at being gray than they are at coloring their hair. "Dyed hair is terribly unattractive on a man," says expert colorist Constance Hartnett.

## "They're just as good-looking and dashing with their gray hair, and they should keep it."

**so why don't men just stay gray?** It's not always vanity that prompts men to color their fading stands. Most insist they're doing it for their careers; they need to maintain a dynamic image in the workplace. Ouidad admits that, in her salon, men account for 25 to 30 percent of her color business, and they are "100 percent career-driven." Suddenly, the young bloods are surrounding them in the office, or the work environment itself may revolve around a very "cool" ethic. Men in the public eye—from celebrities to politicians to CEOs—find it necessary to maintain a youthful, vital appearance. It equates with success.

**taking care of business . . . and themselves** Combe Incorporated, maker of industry leader Just For Men Haircolor, Grecian Formula Haircolor, and Maxim Magazine Color, has long maintained that getting rid of gray is absolutely essential for career success. "It's a more competitive world now, says Michael Wendroff, the company's vice president of men's personal-care marketing," but attitudes are changing, too. A lot of things can enter

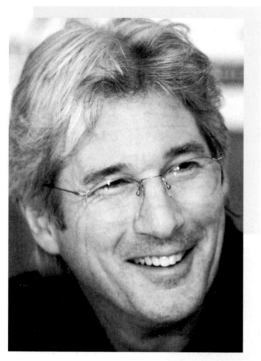

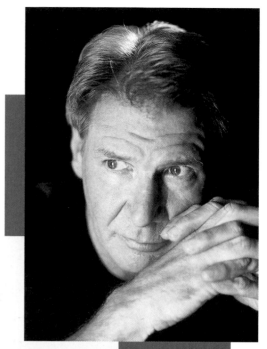

Is it fair? The older men look,
the more gorgeous they get!

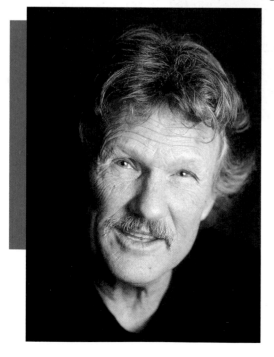

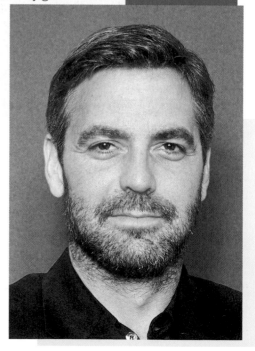

Richard Gere photo © Reuters NewMedia Inc./CORBIS.
All other photos © Peter Freed.

into a man's decision to color his hair, but the whole thing about feeling better about themselves, taking better care of themselves, is really the reason why men feel more comfortable with the idea."

A Roper Starch Worldwide poll, conducted in January 2001, found that more than one-third of the male population polled had either tried coloring their hair or were open to it. According to Wendroff, "Hair coloring is one of the fastest-growing men's grooming categories, faster than men's fragrance and skincare. Men's at-home coloring sales have been increasing consistently over the past ten years, moving into double-digit growth in the last three or four."

So it would seem that everybody's doing it. They're going to the drugstore, they're figuring out what color to buy, and they're hoping for a good match.

### so what's the problem? Can you tell? Many women

insist they always know when a man uses color on his hair. Sometimes, there's a giveaway brassiness, sometimes it has a strange orange cast. The real problem with hair color for men is the warmth, the redness that some products impart. "Women, as they get older and feel they're fading out, are looking for that bright, vibrant tonality," says Chad Murawczyk, president and CEO of Salonclick, makers of MiN Men's Color Match products, available at salons only. "This isn't the right tonality for a man's skin. The shades need to be a little cooler, without being drab or flat. When hair color for men first started, very few companies were formulating color especially for men. There are less than a dozen hair-dye chemists in the United States, and these were the guys who were formulating women's products. If you look at the original swatches for men's hair color, they were all colors that were geared to women."

Enter Just For Men. One of the first products developed to provide safe, easy, and, yes, cool-palette permanent color, well, just for men. Introduced in the mid-1980s, it quickly shot beyond Grecian Formula, the first men's hair-color product in the marketplace, as the coloring of choice. "Over 35 million men have found Just For Men to be trustworthy color," says Michael Wendroff, "and they're very loyal to it, in fact, we have an 80 percent repeater rate. A guy tries it, and he uses it again. So that's our biggest indicator that we're doing something right." After its initial success with shampoo-in hair color, Just For Men came out with a Brush-In Color Gel to shade the trickier areas of mustaches, beards, and sideburns.

The debate between the merits of home color and salon color is as alive for men as it is for women. Which is "better"? It's easier to determine which is the more popular option. Most men, 70 percent, in fact, who color their hair rely on the drugstore brands.

**pick a color, any color?** Do men, unaccustomed to selecting any color that goes near their face, ever know which one to choose? "Medium brown is the biggest-selling drugstore shade because it's perceived as the safest," says Murawczyk. "It's right in the middle, and they figure they can't go wrong. But they can."

Wendroff takes a different view. "Yes, it's the largest-selling shade," he says, "but that's because most men have that color hair." Just For Men makes color selection somewhat foolproof by offering a three-shade "swatch test" on every box. If one of the three colors matches the man's natural hair color, that's the product he should use. If there is any doubt, there are clear, bold instructions to choose a lighter shade. Always the right advice for permanent color products.

But even if it's the right shade to begin with, can't it change and fade? Depends on the formula. "Most off-the-shelf products coat the hair shaft with a metallic sheet of color, and it will continue to build up and look tarry, flat, green. That's what happens; it's an oxidized metallic," says Murawczyk. "Some products give immediate results, but leave a guy with an unnatural-looking color a few weeks out. MiN has a managed regression. We've taken into account how the molecules decouple over time, and the fade-off tone, so it looks natural until his next haircut."

Wendroff says oxidation doesn't apply to Just For Men because there are no metallics in it. "We've reformulated it a number of times over the years as technology has gotten better. It deposits color only on the gray hairs and does not change the natural hair color. So you get a very blended effect until the color grows out. It lasts approximately five to six weeks, and when you use it again, there is no color buildup."

### the get-it-over-with mentality A man who has
never applied a color product to his hair before knows nothing about technique. What he's facing is the emotional baggage that comes from wanting to cover gray. Maybe he's embarrassed about it. Maybe he'll even lock the bathroom door when he does it. But, according to Murawczyk, he won't follow instructions, and he won't get it right.

It's a guy thing. "Every product has a long list of instructions, cautions, peel-off gloves. The man starts to read it and then says the hell with it. So he smudge-smudge-smudges some color on the top and sides of his head. No man knows he has a back of his head. A guy doesn't like to wait for processing time, either, so he hops in the shower too soon and all the color runs down the front and back of his body, which is never a good thing," says Murawczyk. On the other hand, "If it's on too long, it's going to go too dark, and he looks like Elvis."

Both manufacturers of home color and salon color products agree that timing is everything, and must accommodate a man's "hair trigger" when it comes to coloring. MiN Color Match products are designed to work in three to five minutes, in the hands of professionals. Just For Men only takes five minutes of processing time before shampooing out. "It's quick, easy, and goof-proof," says Wendroff. "A man can easily fit it into his regular shower and grooming routine. There's just no mystery about it."

### a matter of degree But what about the nuancing, the
subtle toning, that creates such a natural cover for women's gray? What about the selective shading that allows gray grow-in to go unnoticed for a while? "A man misses out on customized formulation and customized application when he goes to the drugstore," says Murawczyk. "Only the professional can determine the level of gray coverage and the proper tonality. There's no such thing as a 100 percent full-color forty-year-old," he says. "A man hasn't been that since he was twenty-three, and he shouldn't try to be it now. But it's such an individual thing. The professional colorist can take into consideration who he is, how old, how much hair loss he has, *and* how much gray. Fifty percent of good results come from the right product, and

50 percent come from the right application of the product. If the stylist really understands hair color, it's easy."

His last word of advice for men who want to color their hair? "It's like changing the oil in his car. A man should consider it a necessary event, and just get to the salon and do it."

Granted, there are some men who will never feel comfortable in a salon. But that doesn't close the hair-coloring door. Reputable products, good products, are available to them, and the choice of do-it-yourself privacy or salon artistry is theirs to make.

## and then there's the care thing For upkeep,

MiN has formulated a line of hair-care products, developed specifically for men. "Hair is hair," says Chad Murawczyk, "and I take a lot of flack over this. Why should a treatment or styling product be specifically for men? I call ours male-friendly formulations." MiN's line, consisting of a shampoo, called Wash, a conditioner called Rinse, and weightless styling aids that keep color safe, but also tackle things like DHT formation, the follicle-killer responsible for hair loss. "With the right product formulation, you can make a concerted effort to address these problems, and mount a focused attack. It's all about multiple benefits." says Murawczyk. If the man in your life wants to check up on these products, he can visit www.min.com.

Combe Incorporated takes care into account as well. They recommend their Maxim Magazine 2-in-1 Shampoo and Conditioner, especially made for color-treated hair, with fade-resistant UV filters built into the formula.

## the (male) beauty revolution It's happening,

mostly in major cities, but there's a definite shift in grooming attitudes. More and more men are becoming salon savvy. Some borrow a few tricks from their wives' beauty book and go in for color services. But they don't stop there. "You'd be surprised how much men do," says Edward Wilkerson, design director of Lafayette 148. "The other morning, I met a man on the street who told me he has Borghese facials all the time. When I mentioned the weather was really affecting my skin, he recommended a face mask! Women don't know this, but guys are doing the tweezing, the coloring, the facials, and the lifts."

The truth is, men are beginning to mean business in the spa category of beauty services. With the consumer seeking a pampering experience (not to mention a younger look), the skincare/spa industry has blossomed into more than $5 billion industry, incorporating both men's and women's beauty services. As the majority of spa care (57 percent) is offered in full-service beauty salons, it's nothing for a man who is having a massage, facial, or "stress-management" treatment to amble over to the color side of the salon and get something done to his hair.

But even left to his wife's makeup collection, some men are getting pretty sophisticated about adding a little color to their hair, here and there. A woman told me her husband uses two different shades of mascara to tone the gray out of his mustache. Do you use two different colors to tone your eyebrows? Maybe it's time women started taking a page out of their husbands' beauty book!

# hey, you don't have to stay gray

**Ten ways to know if gray doesn't work for you; how to go back; how to go forward.**

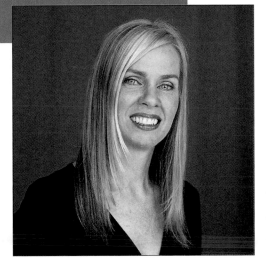

So you did it and you didn't like it. No harm done. Most of us know women who continue to color their hair for life, and look good doing it. Going gray is nature's agenda, but it may not be yours. And that's a personal decision. If you're simply not sure about it, though, it can be a cause of some conflict. You can go back and forth about this for months. Some days you like it, some days you don't. Some days are a draw. Should you "do" something?

This is probably going to be a bigger decision than actually going gray. Trusting your shiny, silvery locks, or your striking white streaks even to semipermanent color is a major commitment. If you're on the fence, my advice is to wait. Let your gray get even better. Still deliberating? Maybe the list below will show you which side of the fence you really *are* on.

## Ten Ways to Know Gray Hair Isn't Working for You

1. You "feel" older and less vital.
2. You look at people who have fully pigmented hair with envy.
3. You don't recognize yourself in pictures, store windows, or the mirror.
4. You've changed your makeup colors, and you still don't feel "bright" enough.
5. You feel your career is in jeopardy.
6. You start worrying about "younger women."
7. You're tired of hearing people tell you to color your hair.
8. You've tried highlighting, lowlighting, and every other kind of lighting, and you still feel there's something more you'd like to do to it.
9. You begin to dress "older."
10. You don't feel like you.

Do you have to experience all ten of them? No. But if only one or two things are bothering you, they're probably easy to fix. The ones that suggest a deeper "attitude" about gray are harder to change, of course. If you think you feel older, and less vital, you'll act older and less vital. You'll probably dress older, as well. It's over, you're saying to yourself. You see how things snowball. If that's what's going on—get away from gray as fast as you can.

Ditto if you feel you've lost out on the career front because of it. It isn't fair, it isn't right, and there are steps you can take to fight it. And ways you can make your gray as impressive as you are. You can boost it a bit, make it more dramatic. Wear it in a sophisticated style that smacks of authority. You can dress well and with confidence. And you can be very good at what you do. But only you know the circumstances of your particular situation. If looking less like an imminent retiree is going to help you keep a job, or get a job, then lose the gray.

If it's just the shock of being gray—catching a glimpse of yourself in a mirror or a window reflection—that will pass. Imagine the shock of seeing yourself suddenly with flaming red hair. Same reaction. It takes a bit of getting used to. Keep this in mind if you opt to "go back" to a color you never were.

And if you're going through a lot of experimentation—changing your makeup colors, your wardrobe palette, having various special effects put into your hair—keep at it until you find the right combination of colors/treat-

> **"It's not for everyone. It takes a lot of confidence. If it's aging, or making you look dumpy, I'd advise a little semipermanent rinse."**
> **Constance Hartnett,**
> **color director, Frédéric Fekkai**

ments that do you justice. When it happens, you'll be delighted with the way you look.

However, if it's all becoming too cumulative—you've got a bad feeling about it, you can't make it work, you just don't feel like yourself—I'm the first to say you should call it quits. It isn't for you. It may be at some other point in your life, but it isn't now. If you've given it your best shot, you don't have to wonder about it. You know.

**going back** So, hey, you don't have to stay gray. And, as Constance Hartnett says, "It's the easiest thing in the world to change." It's a whole lot easier than going gray, that's for

> **"There's an investment involved in taking gray hair back to a darker color. You have to take care of it every two weeks."**
> **Parvin Klein, color director,**
> **John Barrett Salon**

sure. No waiting, no grow-out, no cutting all the colors off. What *is* involved, and you should know this, is frequent visits to the colorist. As you learned in chapter three, those little white roots will start showing up in two weeks' time. If you're going to go significantly darker, the contrast will be so noticeable that it will send you to the salon (or the bottle!) more often than most women.

Revisit "The Root Route" section in chapter three for temporary ways to deal with those pesky gray/white sprouts in between your color applications. Take control of the situation gently, then be patient and wait for your normal appointment. You never want to do too much color, too soon, with a full head of gray hair. It isn't up to it.

### soft shading, subtle color
If you can afford it, it's still wise to put your hair in the hands of a color expert. Someone who can minimize the gray with a multitude of gently harmonizing shades that will blend happily with root growth. This will decrease the frequency of visits to the salon, yet increase the number of services you'll have to have while you are there. Maybe that's a financial toss-up, but you'll have the most natural look, and the longest-lasting color effect.

Remember the nuancing we discussed in chapter three? Go back and see what can be done. And do listen to the advice about not going back to the same shade you were at twenty-three. Discuss a more appropriate tonality with your colorist. Whatever you decide, I beg you not to just dump a color on it and be done with it. You won't be.

### the future looks colorful
Did you know there may be a day when none of us will stay gray? Spontaneous repigmentation has been induced in vitro, using melanocytes taken from gray and white hair follicles. Weird science or not, animals are providing insight into aging hair pigmentation, and reversing the whole process is not beyond the realm of possibility. Scientists have already created a nice crop of glowing green hair for mice by injecting skin grafts with a glowing green gene, of course. Researchers have also genetically modified albino rats and mice by altering a tyrosinase mutation in a hair follicle gene. Tyrosinase, if you'll remember from chapter five, is the enzyme involved in the synthesis of melanin. The result? Pure white mice sprouted black hair. Although this is the first step toward a genetic treatment for graying hair, it's only that. They have yet to come up with a variety of colors. Which genes cause which pigments is still unknown.

So if glowing green or black isn't your shade, hang on. There's a lot going on in the world of follicular gene therapy. Although, admittedly, nearly *all* your hair follicles would have to be modified to create a full head of nongray hair, so maybe you shouldn't kiss your salon good-bye quite yet.

But there is encouraging news on other fronts. Hair loss may one day be reversed this way. Scientists haven't found the balding gene yet, but hair-graft transplants may benefit from gene manipulation and be prompted to grow more hair. Genes encased in liposomes—you know liposomes from certain skincare products—have also been massaged onto follicles, with varying results. But one day we may just have a moisturizer-like product that we can apply to our hair, and poof! no more female pattern baldness. We aren't there yet. And the jury is still out about converting what works on mice to men. Or women, for that matter. If safe repigmentation and regrowth techniques become available as simple cosmetics, you'll simply have another alternative to going gray, another thing to try, another thing to do. Will it be worth it? That's up to you. It depends on how great you feel, how great you look, as your hair goes through the most natural transition in the world.

In the meantime, if you wish to recolor your gray hair, be thankful you have a wide selection of safe products and services from which choose. Be thankful there are expert colorists who can help you do it subtly and beautifully. And, most of all, no matter what shade you choose to be—a glorious gray or an artful color—be thankful for yourself!

# afterword

Something funny started happening as I was writing this book. I began to see more and more women at some stage of graying. I couldn't go out without spotting at least three or four. I couldn't go to a social event without making a beeline for a great-looking gray. Very often, if I were walking, I would change my path so I could approach a silvery stranger, learn her secrets. At other times, a woman would be engaged in conversation, or otherwise inaccessible. She'd be in a car, or I'd be in a cab passing by. I would consider stopping the cab and jumping out, but she would turn a corner and disappear. These near-misses frustrated me. It seemed as if there were millions of great grays all around me, and I couldn't get to them all.

I like to think this book is one way to "get to them all." But as I prepared to deliver it to the publisher, I kept seeing more and more women with gray hair. The urge to run after them, to stop them in their tracks continued. And the names, the lists of women whom people wanted me to "talk to" kept coming. Oh, you must include my sister/mother/niece/aunt/coworker/friend—she's great. And I wanted to, I really wanted to. But, deadlines being deadlines, I had to stop.

But it doesn't stop. Look at the generation just coming into its own glorious "grayhood." A boomer turns fifty every seven seconds? They turn gray faster than that. I may have missed someone who should be in this book, who has every right to be in it. Something in me said, "*Wait,* wait for them." But publishers have schedules, and the most important thing was to get this book into print.

Just know, whenever you read this book, I'll probably still be stopping a "great gray" on the street and talking to her about her hair. I'll probably wish that she were in this book. And maybe, one day, I'll even stop you. Don't be surprised.

In the meantime, enjoy your new color, and remember—this is just the beginning.

# acknowledgments

Putting a book like this together takes a real cast of characters. I'm inclined to say "roll credits" as I pass out thanks to one and all. First, and without whom, there would be no book on gray hair, my literary agent Judith Riven. I'll admit: It was all her idea. She'll admit: It took some convincing to get me to do it. Okay, I was naïve and nongray when the book began. And then I started talking to women. Meeting so many terrific, confident, successful women that I was swept up in their joy of being gray and being great.

Committed to the project, I began interviewing a score of photographers. But it was Judith Riven again who found the plum: Peter Freed. Best known for celebrity portraits of top-caliber stars and entertainment professionals like Tom Cruise, Julia Roberts, Hugh Grant, Harrison Ford, Reese Witherspoon, Liza Minelli, Siguorney Weaver, Robert De Niro, and so many other well-known names in the arts, business, and political fields, he seemed unapproachable. He wasn't. Peter finds beauty in every woman, and he was taken by the subject of this book. At every turn, he was a true collaborator and friend. His easy style instantly relaxed women unaccustomed to modeling so they could have fun in front of the camera, abetted by Peter's transformational lighting and loving lens.

Hair. I thought it would be wonderful to have one of the best salons in New York City work with us on styling and coloring. I couldn't have wished for better than the Minardi Salon. Owners Beth and Carmine Minardi were as captivated by the topic as we all were. Known to women across the country through countless editorial credits, and ask-the-experts advice in numerous magazines, the Minardis are equally well known to people in the industry. Conducting seminars the world over, they're the hair professional's professionals, and widely respected in their field. With a clientele that includes celebrities and royalty alike, Beth and Carmine are also in demand for creating the perfect coifs (and color) for movie shoots. So I was thrilled when they volunteered time, staff, and expertise for our shoots. Through many, many hours of cutting, styling, and coloring, every artist and staff member demonstrated superior professional skills, as well as a great deal of tender loving care. And, if you've ever tried to schedule hair appointments for a multitude of women, you'll know that Zoe and Carol deserve special medals!

All that was left was wardrobe. My longtime friend and fashion industry legend Gloria Gelfand thought the book a "brilliant" idea, and she put me in touch with Lafayette 148 New York. By this time, enthusiasm for the project didn't surprise me in the least. Deirdre Quinn, president of the well-known bridge line, assured me of full cooperation, and a team of collection experts, led by Aileen Dresner, executive vice president, spent many hours fitting and selecting appropriate styles for every woman we would photograph. They managed to make each appointment a pampering experience, and notes of thanks would arrive promptly after a fitting. Thank you all for being gracious, professional, and comforting to everyone—including the author! And a million more thanks to Edward Wilkerson for designing the clothes that allow women to feel beautiful, professional, and simply "right."

Everything was falling into place, but there was so much more. So many more people to contact, so much information to get. And so many people in the know who were willing to help me. From major cosmetics and skincare executives to public relations people in various fields. From dermatologists to psychologists. From top fashion executives at Neiman Marcus, Joan Kaner and Sandra Wilson, to boutique retailers like Noemi Goureau at Fopp's, Paris and Marilyn Ko of Che Che New York. From well-known jewelry manufacturers to women who crafted their own. The list went on and on.

Special thanks to those in the business of beauty who had the vision to realize the importance of women others chose to overlook. In their thinking, there was no question, no hesitation, no second-guessing about the beauty of women with gray in their hair, or the viability of this market. Particularly, Sally Sussman and Melissa Bedolis Cattanach at Estée Lauder; Michael Trese, Susan Bang, and Sarah Corrao at L'Oréal; Caroline Pieper-Vogt and Jenny D'Adamo at Clarins.

And then, suddenly, at the shoots, magic did indeed happen. Due in no small part to Jennifer Wobito, makeup artist extraordinare. Her special talent is achieving a naturally beautiful look; never "made-up," never artificial. Most of the women were so delighted they wanted to know—specifically—the products and the colors she used. Jennifer would diligently e-mail lists to those who asked, going above and beyond makeup artist duty. In addition, her good spirit and snappy attitude kept us all laughing. "Tweak?" she would say. "You want me to *tweak?*" A makeup artist who has done everything from fashion shoots to celebrities to weddings, Jennifer much prefers working on "real women."

Many thanks to Trish Todd, editor in chief of trade paperbacks at Simon & Schuster, who believed in this book from the beginning, and had the determination, negotiating skill, and patience to bring it in. And to my editor, Beth Wareham, who wanted to do it even if it meant switching imprints. Without her great insight and kind editing, the book would never have had the "cut and blow-dry" it needed. She was totally in tune with what we hoped this book would be, and her enthusiasm and winning personality made it all that much easier. Thanks also to Beth's very smart publishing associate, Rica Buxbaum Allannic, who found the right answers and humored me at the right time.

Others provided creative and critical assistance at the right time, solving problems, lending their talents, and opening doors. I would probably still be stuck in chapter two without the help of my longtime friends Susan Rafaj, Mary Lou Sinatra, and art director/angel John Collier. And, on the other side of the Atlantic, Marion Beckmann, Ina, and Oliver. And thanks to my "stringers," Linn Joslyn and Christine Hermann for gathering quotes from the distaff side.

But none of this would have happened without the women I call my "Great Grays," my GGs. Whether they had a few paltry salty strands, or a head full of glorious white hair; whether they were members of the very first panel discussion, or talked to me at great length on the phone; whether they met me for an interview, or took time out of their busy days to be washed/cut/blow-dried/colored/made up/photographed, they were all my inspiration. And I thank them for sharing their thoughts and time. I hope I have formed many lasting friendships among this group of remarkable women. And so, while I would like to thank each and every person individually for helping me create the first beauty book devoted to women who choose to be pigment-free, it's best to just *roll credits.*

## The GGs

Sherrill Adams
Deborah Aiges
Leni Anders
Jennie Benard
Janice Bryant
Rita Citrin
Liz Cullumber
Penn Curran
Pat Cush
Francine Matalon-Degni
Jamie deRoy
Mary Louise Farrell
Alice Feder
Shirley Feder
Patricia Flannery

Ellen Fox
Carmine Fuentes
Lanell Goodman
Irene Breslaw Grapel
Christine Herman
Setsuka Nagata Ikeda
Joan Kaner
Marilyn Ko
Ruth Lawson
Chazz Levi
Silvia Maginnis
Dr. Patricia Moscou
Angela Muriel
Nancy Ozelli
Joan Parks

JoAnne Pinto
Amy Robinson
Ruth Robinson
Dara Roche
Ilene Rosen
Kim Sava
Marilyn Sokol
Mia Fonssagrives Solow
Carol Tanenbaum
Dr. Anne-Renée Testa
Amy Trakinski
Rita Wells
Peri Wolfman

## Hair

**Minardi Salon**
Beth Minardi, color director
Carmine Minardi, style director

*Stylists*
Shannon Briggs
Sachi Fukumoto
Tammy Laimos
Melanie Moses
Maria Perrotti

*Colorists*
Kenneth Bradley
Renée Rockefeller

*Shoot Scheduling*
Zoe Stark

*Appointment Staff*
Heather Dolinsky
Sonny Shirley
Wendy Rasher

*Scheduling Management*
Carol Krisulevicz

**Frédéric Fekkai Salon**
Constance Hartnett, color director
**John Barrett Salon**
John Barrett
Deborah Hardwick
Parvin Klein, color director

Claire Bruno, industry consultant
Robert Oppenheim, former chairman and president, Clairol Professional Products Division; founder and board member, American Beauty Association
Kevin Maple, Kevin Maple Salon, Southampton
Chad Murawczyk, president and CEO Salonclick, LLC
Ouidad, "Queen of Curl," and author of *Curl Talk*
Michael Wendroff, vice president, Men's Personal Care Marketing, Combe, Inc.

## Makeup
Laura Hess from FACE
Tammy Laimos
Jennifer Wobito

## Beauty and Skin Care
Susan Bang, director, public relations, L'Oréal
Julie Berman, director, public relations, Clinique
Melissa Bedolis Cattanach, vice president, global communications, Estée Lauder Companies
Carol Cefaratti, chief aesthetician, Ellen Lange Skin Science

Sarah Corrao, public relations manager, L'Oréal
Jenny D'Adamo, director makeup and fragrance marketing, Clarins Brand
Kathy Dwyer, founder and CEO, Skinklinic
Janet Carlson Freed, beauty and health director, *Town & Country*
Lois Joy Johnson, beauty and fashion director, *More* magazine
Ellen Lange, president and founder, Ellen Lange Skin Science
Eileen Paley, senior vice president, marketing/product development, Georgette Klinger
Caroline Pieper-Vogt, vice president, marketing, Clarins
Sally Sussman, senior vice president, communications, the Estée Lauder Companies
Michael Trese, vice president, public relations, L'Oréal
Cheryl Vitali, consultant

Dr. Daniel Maes, vice president, research and development, Estée Lauder Worldwide
Dr. Dennis Gross, dermatologist and founder, MD Skincare
Dr. Lydia M. Evans, consulting dermatologist, L'Oréal
Dr. Jonathan B. Levine, D.M.D. and founder, GoSmile

## Psychologists
Dr. Patricia Moscou
Dr. Anne-Renée Testa

# acknowledgments

## Fashion

**Lafayette 148 New York**
Deirdre Quinn, president
Edward Wilkerson, design director
Aileen Dresner, executive vice
  president
Deirdre Byrne
King Chong
Meaghan Ryan
Frankie Yan

Gloria Gelfand
Joan Kaner, senior vice president,
  fashion director, Neiman Marcus
Sandra Wilson, accessories fashion
  director, senior fashion editor,
  Neiman Marcus
Licia Hahn
Betty Halbreich, Bergdorf Goodman
  "Solutions," and author of *Secrets
  of a Fashion Therapist*

## Jewelry

Stephen Dweck
Ippolita
Che Che New York
Mia Fonssagrives Solow at Gumps
Deborah Aiges
Georgina Saccone for Southern
  Artisans

## Marketing and Public Relations

Susan M. Rafaj Marketing
  Services Inc.
Tally Boniface, Bratskeir & Company
Amy Metrick, Ketchum
Kristen Laney, Ketchum
Simone B. Hoffman, Wish List
  Consulting Group
Judy Katz, theatrical publicist
Maria Yatskova, public relations, New
  York Philharmonic

## Locations

Linn Hughes, for her beautiful loft
Hank Meiman, theatre manager, West
  Bank Café

## Illustrations and Graphics

Graham Anderson
John Collier

## Panel Session Photography

Ed Goldman

## Celebrity Photography

Joan Marcus
Reuters NewMedia

## Peter's Assistants

Heather Blanton
Adrianna Lopez
Rob Stoddard
Stacy Zarin

232

# index

# about the author

A former marketing director of *Vogue* and promotion director of *Seventeen,* DIANA LEWIS JEWELL knows the business of bringing beauty and fashion alive for the consumer. She has written seven nonfiction books, including the longest-selling beauty book of all time, *Making Up by Rex.* As one of New York's best-known freelance copywriters, her clients compose a virtual who's who of the leading names in cosmetics and skincare, fragrances, and international fashion. Diana lives in Manhattan and Southampton with her husband, David, and is currently, very happily, going gray.